Prenatal Testing for Late-Onset Neurogenetic Diseases

Prenatal Testing for Late-Onset Neurogenetic Diseases

Edited by

G. Evers-Kiebooms
Center for Human Genetics, University of Leuven, Belgium

M. W. Zoeteweij
Clinical Genetics Centre, Academic Hospital Leiden, The Netherlands

P. S. Harper
Institute of Medical Genetics, University of Wales College of Medicine, Cardiff, UK

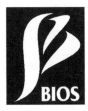

First published 2002

A CIP catalogue record for this book is available from the British Library.

ISBN 1 85996 019 7

BIOS Scientific Publishers Ltd
9 Newtec Place, Magdalen Road, Oxford OX4 1RE, UK
Tel. +44 (0)1865 726286. Fax +44 (0)1865 246823
World Wide Web home page: http://www.bios.co.uk/

Distributed exclusively in the United States, its dependent territories, Canada, Mexico, Central and South America, and the Carribean by Springer-Verlag New York Inc., 175 Fifth Avenue, New York, USA, by arrangement with BIOS Scientific Publishers Ltd., 9 Newtec Place, Magdalen Road, Oxford OX4 1RE, UK

Production Editor: Andrea Bosher.
Typeset by Kolam Information Service, Pondicherry, India
Printed by Cromwell Press, Trowbridge, UK

Contents

Abbreviations

ADCA	autosomal dominant cerebellar ataxias
AMDTG	Ataxia Molecular Diagnostic Testing Group
ART	assisted reproductive technology
CVB	chorionic villus biopsy
EC	European Commission
FSH	follicle-stimulating hormone
GIFT	gamete intrafallopian transfer
hCG	human chorionic gonadotrophin
HD	Huntington's disease
ICSI	intracytoplasmic sperm injection
IVF	in vitro fertilization
LH	luteinizing hormone
PGD	preimplantation genetic diagnosis
RCNRT	Royal Commission on New Reproductive Technologies
US HD GTG	United States Huntington Disease Genetic Testing Group
WFNRHD	World Federation of the Neurology Research Group on Huntington's disease

Contributors

Craufurd, D. MD, Psychiatrist, Academic Unit of Medical Genetics and Regional Genetic Service, St. Mary's Hospital, Manchester, UK

de Die, C. MD, PhD, Clinical Geneticist, Clinical Genetics Center, Maastricht, The Netherlands

de Wert, G. PhD in Ethics, Institute for Bioethics, Universiteit Maastricht, Maastricht, The Netherlands

Decruyenaere, M. PhD in Psychology, Psychosocial Genetics Unit, Center for Human Genetics, Leuven, Belgium

Desmet, C. Master in Law, Center for Biomedical Ethics and Law, Leuven, Belgium

Dürr, A. MD, Clinical Geneticist, Département de Génétique, Cytogénétique et Embryologie, Hôpital de la Salpêtrière, Paris, France

Evers-Kiebooms, G. Prof., PhD in Psychology, Psychosocial Genetics Unit, Center for Human Genetics, Leuven, Belgium

Feingold, J. MD, Clinical Geneticist, Département de Génétique, Cytogénétique et Embryologie, Hôpital de la Salpêtrière, Paris, France

Geraedts, J.P.M. Prof., PhD in Molecular Genetics, Universiteit Maastricht, Maastricht, The Netherlands

Harper, P.S. Prof., MD, Physician, Clinical Geneticist, Institute of Medical Genetics, Cardiff, UK

Harper, R. MD, Psychiatrist, Institute of Medical Genetics, Cardiff, UK

Heurckmans, N. Clinical Psychologist, Free University of Brussels (VUB), Brussels, Belgium

Jacopini, G. PhD in Psychology, Istituto di Psicologia, Consiglio Nazionale Ricerche, Rome, Italy

Laccone, F. MD, PhD, Geneticist, Institut für Humangenetik, Göttingen, Germany

Liebaers, I. Prof., MD, PhD, Clinical Geneticist, Centre for Medical Genetics, Free Brussels University (VUB), Brussels, Belgium

Nance, M.A. MD, Neurologist, Hennepin County Medical Center, St. Louis Park, MN 55426, USA

Nys, H. Prof., PhD in Law, Center for Biomedical Ethics and Law, Leuven, Belgium

Nys, K. Clinical Psychologist, Psychosocial Genetics Unit, Center for Human Genetics, Leuven, Belgium

Romeo-Casabona, C.M. Prof., PhD in Law, Catedra de Derechoy Genome Humano, Universidad de Deusto, Bilbao, Spain

Simpson, S.A. MD, Clinical Geneticist, Clinical Genetics, Grampian University Hospital, Aberdeen, UK

Sørensen, S.A. Prof., MD, PhD, Clinical Geneticist, Department of Medical Genetics, The Panum Institute, University of Copenhagen, Copenhagen, Denmark

Varkevisser, K. MD, European Huntington Association

Watkin, S. President of the International Huntington Association

Yapijakis, C. DMD, MS, PhD Neurogeneticist, Department of Neurology, University of Athens Medical School, Athens, Greece

Zoeteweij, M.W. PhD in Psychology, Department of Clinical Genetics, Leiden, The Netherlands

Preface

This book examines the clinical, psychological, social, ethical and legal complexity of prenatal testing and preimplantation genetic diagnosis for Huntington's disease and other late-onset neurogenetic diseases. Multidisciplinarity is a major characteristic of the book and special attention has been paid to the family's perspective. All the authors of this book have been intensively involved in issues related to predictive and prenatal testing in practice and/or research for many years. The two chapters with several vivid case presentations are of irreplaceable value; the book would be seriously incomplete without them and would lose a special quality of relevance and individual involvement.

About 15 years ago predictive testing and prenatal testing for Huntington's disease became feasible. This was a new challenge for families and professionals. In the meantime many predictive and prenatal tests have been performed, initially indirectly by DNA-linkage and since 1993 by direct mutation analysis. Moreover, Huntington's disease has been a model for dealing with predictive and prenatal testing for other late-onset neurogenetic diseases.

This book arose from a European collaborative study and from a European BIOMED meeting held in Leuven, Belgium, in November 2000. The European collaborative study focussed on Huntington's disease and involved professionals from genetic centers in six different European countries, an expert in the legal aspects of genetic testing, an expert in the ethical aspects of genetic testing and a participant from the European Huntington Association. This study was carried out in the context of a European Commission (EC) funded BIOMED-project. The European meeting had a broader scope: an extension was made to preimplantation genetic diagnosis, to other late-onset neurogenetic diseases and to other European countries. A considerable number of chapters in the book are extensive elaborations of one or more presentations during the meeting in Leuven. Others, including a chapter about predictive and prenatal testing for neurogenetic diseases in North America, have been written exclusively for this book without any link to the European project or meeting.

This book gives more insight in the complexity of prenatal testing for late-onset neurogenetic disease. We hope that it will result in improving the professional care and support for all families who are confronted with the burden imposed by late-onset neurogenetic disease.

Gerry Evers-Kiebooms

Acknowledgements

The production of this volume represents the collective achievement of the three editors, all contributors and many other people. It would have been impossible without the funding of the European BIOMED-project No. ERB BMH4–CT98–3926. Thanks to the EC funding a systematic European collaborative study could be undertaken and a multidisciplinary European meeting with invited speakers and invited participants from most EC-countries could be organised. In particular the latter resulted in the initiative to produce this book with a broader scope. Looking back on the past 5 years I would particularly like to thank my secretary, Narcisse Opdekamp, for her important role throughout the project, the meeting and the realisation of this volume. Very special gratitude is extended to my husband, my sons and my family...they know why.

Gerry Evers-Kiebooms

Introduction
Complexity of predictive and prenatal testing for neurogenetic late-onset diseases

Gerry Evers-Kiebooms

1. Some introductory remarks about predictive and prenatal testing for late-onset neurogenetic disease

When predictive testing and prenatal testing for Huntington's disease (HD) became a reality, about 15 years ago, this was an important milestone in medical history and a new challenge for families and professionals. Since then, many predictive and prenatal tests have been performed, initially indirectly using DNA linkage and since 1993 using direct mutation analysis. Moreover, increasing knowledge about the human genome has resulted in the availability of predictive tests and prenatal tests for other neurogenetic diseases and hereditary cancers. The topic of genetic testing for hereditary cancers is beyond the scope of this book, in which the focus is on prenatal testing for neurogenetic late-onset disease. However, predictive testing for neurogenetic late-onset disease receives attention in several chapters of this book because of its special relationship with prenatal testing.

   Predictive tests for late-onset neurogenetic diseases provide information about 'an asymptomatic person's future health status regarding a specific disease'. This type of test is very different from most other medical examinations, which usually concern 'a person's present health status'. For this reason, it is essential to keep in mind that an asymptomatic person with the mutant gene will stay healthy for an unpredictable number of years: the test

Prenatal Testing for Late-Onset Neurogenetic Diseases, edited by G. Evers-Kiebooms,
M. W. Zoeteweij and P. S. Harper
©2002 BIOS Scientific Publishers Ltd, Oxford

really concerns *pre*symptomatic diagnosis. Moreover, an individual prediction about the exact age at onset, the specific symptoms or the course of the disease is impossible. In other words, a degree of uncertainty persists. The difference between predictive tests (detecting the presence or absence of a mutation but not the presence or absence of symptoms) and examinations aimed at early diagnosis (detecting early symptoms of the disease) is so huge that society has not yet sufficiently adapted to this situation. This is true for potential test applicants and healthcare professionals, as well as for other groups in society. This lack of awareness may create a situation wherein persons with an unfavourable predictive test result may be considered as affected in a too early stage (in the presymptomatic stage), a risk that should not be neglected. Predictive tests for late-onset neurogenetic diseases have far-reaching implications for the test applicants, their family and for society (Harper and Clarke, 1997). The above-mentioned characteristics of predictive testing and the fact that they lead to a new status or psychological identity have important consequences for the context in which these tests should be offered as a clinical service. It is of the utmost importance that a real choice about having or not having a predictive test is safeguarded. This choice should be a well-informed, free and personal decision of the test applicant without external pressure. This is the more true because there usually is no medical reason at all to perform this type of test. The availability of predictive tests gives informed people the choice 'to know' or 'not to know', a decision with important short-, mid- and long-term consequences. Because of the particular nature of predictive tests for (currently) untreatable late-onset diseases, a large amount of international debate and consultation preceded the implementation of the first predictive and prenatal tests for HD in clinical practice. The guidelines elaborated by the International Huntington Association and the World Federation of Neurology (1994) have in the meantime been used as a model for predictive testing for other neurogenetic diseases, in particular the autosomal dominant form of amyotrophic lateral sclerosis (Rowland and Shneider, 2001) and autosomal dominant cerebellar ataxias (Chapter 11).

This book focuses on prenatal testing (full prenatal diagnosis, prenatal exclusion testing and preimplantation genetic diagnosis) within the context of the complex process of reproductive decision-making that people at increased genetic risk for a late-onset neurogenetic disease face. The editors and authors of this book are professionals who have all been very actively involved, some of them long before the availability of predictive DNA testing, in HD and other neurogenetic diseases in practice and/or research. Multidisciplinarity is a major characteristic of this book: the chapters cover clinical, psychological, social, ethical and legal aspects of prenatal testing for neurogenetic late-onset diseases. Moreover, the family's perspective is an integral part of this book.

In the following section, the need for a multidisciplinary approach to predictive testing for HD is stressed. Thereafter, the uptake for predictive testing and the factors involved in decision-making to have or not have a predictive test for HD are briefly reviewed. The last section introduces the topics that are discussed in this book.

2. Predictive testing for Huntington's disease: the elaboration of careful protocols and the need for a multidisciplinary approach

Huntington's disease (HD) is a currently untreatable progressive neuropsychiatric disorder, characterized by involuntary movements, neuropsychological defects and personality changes. The mean age at onset is about 40 years. Symptoms progress slowly with death occurring an average of 15 years after disease onset. Huntington's disease is inherited as an autosomal dominant trait, with the gene localized on the short arm of chromosome 4. In March 1993, the Huntington gene was isolated containing an expanded and unstable trinucleotide repeat (CAG) in HD patients (Huntington's Disease Collaborative Research Group, 1993). The localization and subsequent identification of the gene resulted in the offer of a predictive DNA test to asymptomatic persons belonging to families with HD. In a recent paper, Harper et al. (2000), on behalf of the UK Huntington's Disease Prediction Consortium, stated that 'the normal range was classified as up to 30 repeats, with 39 or more repeats as abnormal, the small intervening number being considered as "equivocal"' (p. 568). Persons with a predictive test result in the latter category are also called persons with an intermediate allele; this result is quite exceptional ($\pm 1.5\%$ of the persons with a predictive test in the UK during the period 1988–1997).

Predictive test protocols have been carefully established because the potential pitfalls were widely recognized before offering predictive testing as a clinical service. Internationally agreed guidelines have been issued. They are aimed at protecting test applicants and at assisting clinicians, geneticists and ethical committees, as well as lay organizations, to resolve difficulties arising from the application of the test. One of the guidelines precludes predictive testing of children on parental request: this type of test with far-reaching consequences should not be carried out until the child has reached legal majority and is competent to make his or her own free decision. It is essential to respect the child's right not to know. However, some adolescents who are actively requesting HD predictive testing of their own accord pose a difficult dilemma. In this situation, adequate criteria are needed to assess the adolescent's competence to make a decision about a predictive test.

Predictive test requests are often approached by a multidisciplinary team consisting of a clinical geneticist, a psychologist, a neurologist and/or a social worker or genetic nurse. The number of professionals involved may differ from one centre to another. During the pretest counselling sessions, full information is provided on HD and on the predictive test. The role and psychological meaning of the disease and the test during the life course of the testee are explored. It is the main aim of these pretest counselling sessions to help people to give sufficient time to reflection, to develop a scenario of their life after a favourable test result, after an unfavourable test result or without having a predictive test and to make a free informed decision about having or not having a predictive test. After the disclosure of the predictive test result, short- and long-term emotional and social support is systematically provided during follow-up counselling sessions. The partner of the test applicant is encouraged to participate in all pretest and post-test counselling sessions. The number of pretest counselling sessions, as well as the post-test follow-up, in particular the long-term follow-up may differ from one country to another as well from one centre to another within the same country.

3. Uptake for predictive testing and prenatal testing for Huntington's disease

All over the world the proportion of persons who have applied for predictive testing is smaller than expected based on intentions and attitudes before the availability of the test: the uptake rate varies between 5 and 20% (cf. Craufurd et al., 1989; Evers-Kiebooms and Decruyenaere, 1998; Quaid and Morris, 1993; Tibben et al., 1992; Tyler et al., 1992).

In the genetic centre in Leuven, uptake was calculated for all sibships with at least one individual with a prior risk of 50%, who had applied for predictive testing since the start of the test programme at the end of 1987 (Evers-Kiebooms and Decruyenaere, 1998). Of all the potential test candidates in these sibships (i.e. all non-affected living adults), about 1 in 4 had been tested. This figure is the upper limit and probably a considerable overestimation of the real uptake in the total group of individuals with a 50% risk; indeed in many sibships nobody requests predictive testing. The survey in siblings of persons who applied for predictive testing in Leuven clearly revealed that a predictive test request is an individual rather than a familial matter. It is very hard to unravel why only a minority of individuals at risk have chosen to be tested, while most others prefer not to be tested. It is obvious that demographic variables play hardly any part in the decision. The perceived susceptibility and severity are also rather similar in tested and untested individuals. Personality profile and individual coping style seem to be the key factors in the decision to be tested. Here, it is important to draw attention to the fact that the group of untested persons is very heterogeneous and consists of at least two different subgroups: a first group who has deliberately chosen not to take the test and who copes well with the uncertainty and a second group with avoidance behaviour regarding the disease, the risk and the test.

Decruyenaere et al. (1997) assessed the perceived benefits or reasons for taking the test and the perceived barriers against taking the test in tested and untested persons belonging to the same sibships. The most important benefits or reasons for taking the test are: the need for certainty or relief from uncertainty, making reproductive decisions, informing their children about their risk for HD and making decisions on practical matters (financial, employment). Important barriers against the test are: the anticipated inability to cope with a bad test result, the feeling that important decisions do not have to depend on a test result, being happier not knowing rather than having to cope with the certainty of a bad result, the lack of a treatment, concern about the reaction of their children and partner. The reported benefits and barriers have been confirmed in other studies (Quaid and Morris, 1993; Van der Steenstraten *et al.*, 1994). In some countries, concern about life insurance is an additional barrier to taking the test (Harper, 1996). Of course the motivation to have or not have a predictive test is very complex, (there is often more than one reason or motive) and consists of conscious and unconscious motives. It is important to keep in mind that in most surveys or other studies only the conscious motives expressed or indicated by the persons at risk for HD are taken into account. In most centres around the world that have reported their data, the two major motives for requesting predictive testing are 'certainty for the own future' and 'family planning'. For a review on the impact of predictive testing on the psychological well-being of testees and their family we refer to Evers-Kiebooms *et al.* (2000). With respect to family planning, the findings in many centres around the world (Adam *et al.*, 1993; Decruyenaere *et al.*, 1997; Evers-Kiebooms *et al.*, 1996; Schulman *et al.*, 1996; Tolmie *et al.*, 1995; Tyler *et al.*, 1990) illustrate that carriers of the HD mutation with a desire for children are confronted with new decision difficulties and an additional emotional burden. They have the following options: refraining from having children, taking the risk of having a child with the Huntington mutation, using prenatal diagnosis, artificial insemination with donor sperm, IVF with donor eggs and, more recently in a small number of centres around the world, preimplantation genetic diagnosis (PGD). This book explicitly discusses the use of prenatal testing and PGD for HD and to a lesser extent for other neurogenetic diseases. When considering prenatal testing for late-onset disease, it is important to make a distinction between 'full prenatal testing' aimed at obtaining all the available information concerning the specific late-onset disease (before 1993 by DNA linkage, thereafter by direct mutation analysis) and 'prenatal exclusion testing' aimed at determining whether the fetus has the same genetic risk as the asymptomatic at-risk parent belonging to the Huntington family or no risk for HD. In the latter case, one determines whether the fetus inherited a chromosome 4 from the affected grandparent or from the partner of the affected grandparent and no information is given about the genetic status of the at-risk parent. Initially, prenatal exclusion testing was introduced mainly as an option for couples with an uninformative family structure, for whom predictive testing was impossible because of technical limitations. Following identification of the gene in 1993 the option continued to be offered to at-risk persons who did not want a predictive test to know their own status but who wanted to prevent the transmission of the disease to their children.

Results of a survey assessing the uptake of prenatal testing for HD worldwide, carried out in close collaboration with the World Federation of the Neurology Research Group on Huntington's Disease, revealed that the uptake of prenatal testing is low, but that the results largely vary between different countries and between different centres within a country (Evers-Kiebooms, 1997). The prediction of Hayden *et al.* (1995) that the demand for prenatal testing would further decrease in the future because of the optimism about a potential treatment has come true in some countries. Recently, Hayden (2001) reported that not a single prenatal test for HD has been performed in British Columbia during the past 5 years. The uptake for prenatal testing in Europe and in North America is discussed in several chapters in this book. Hereby, specific attention is also paid to the difficult situation that arises when parents decide to continue the pregnancy when the fetus is a carrier of the Huntington mutation. Indeed the child to be born may later in his life be harmed by this information. It cannot be excluded that the known carrier status may have a negative impact on the child's upbringing: either by spoiling or overprotecting or by neglecting the child. Moreover the child's right not to know is already violated before his birth. All these issues should receive attention during counselling before the parents engage in a pregnancy with prenatal diagnosis.

4. The scope of this book

To obtain more insight into the psychosocial, ethical and legal complexity of prenatal testing for HD, a European collaborative, multidisciplinary study was set up with participants from several genetic centres, one with expertise in the legal aspects of genetic testing, one with expertise in the ethical aspects of genetic testing and one from the European Huntington Association. This study was carried out in the context of a European Commission (EC) funded project (BIOMED-project No ERB BMH4–CT98–3926). Notwithstanding the fact that this European project was the starting point for this book, the scope of this book is wider and several experts who did not participate in the project have been invited to contribute to this book either as the author of an entire chapter or as a co-author responsible for part of a chapter.

Because the European project was the origin of this book and because it eventually resulted in about half of the chapters in the book, the objectives of the European project are presented first.

(i) Creating a detailed picture of prenatal testing for HD (full prenatal testing as well as exclusion prenatal testing) in six countries in different parts of the European Community (Belgium, France, Italy, Greece, The Netherlands, UK).

(ii) Obtaining insight into the reproductive decision-making of carriers of the Huntington mutation who are at reproductive age compared with non-carriers and evaluating the uptake of prenatal testing for the former group in the seven genetic centres involved in the project (Aberdeen, Athens, Cardiff, Leuven, Leiden, Paris, Rome).

(iii) Delineating the factors that explain the differences in uptake for prenatal testing as well as differences in reproductive history following predictive testing.

(iv) Analysing the ethical and legal implications of prenatal testing for HD.

(v) Stimulating discussion about the findings between professionals from different disciplines (medical, ethical, psychological and legal) and HD associations.

(vi) Using the experience gained from HD to construct a model system for the complex ethical, psychosocial and legal aspects of prenatal testing and PGD in other late-onset neurogenetic diseases.

Six chapters in this book (2, 3, 4, 6, 9, 10) are directly related to the European project. Chapter 2 by Jacopini *et al.* is aimed at giving a salient and real-life picture of prenatal testing by means of case presentations of prenatal testing in three European countries. All names and some irrelevant details have been changed to guarantee the anonymity of the couples who had one or more prenatal tests. Chapter 3 by Zoeteweij *et al.* presents the results of the European collaborative study on the series of prenatal tests in the seven participating centres since the start of their programme. Each of the participating centres additionally provided data for the other centres in their country (Belgium, France, Italy, Greece, The Netherlands and UK). In this chapter the phenomenon of repeated prenatal testing receives special attention. Chapter 4 by Evers-Kiebooms *et al.* presents the results of another part of the European collaborative study, namely the impact of the predictive test result upon subsequent reproduction, including the uptake for prenatal testing in the group of carriers of the Huntington mutation. Chapter 6 by Nys *et al.* deals mainly with those legal aspects of prenatal testing that are most relevant for prenatal testing for late-onset neurogenetic diseases. The discussion of the legal protection of the unborn child and the termination of pregnancy is followed by a section on the rights of the parents and the child. The chapter ends with comments on the liability of the geneticist for wrongful birth and wrongful life. Chapter 9 by de Wert starts with reflections on non-directiveness and discusses the ethical aspects of the various methods of prenatal testing and PGD. It also sketches some implications for and dilemmas regarding prenatal testing for other late-onset diseases. Chapter 10 by Watkin and Varkevisser gives a lay perspective on dilemmas and problems facing Huntington families in the context of prenatal testing and PGD. It clearly stresses the wide variety of opinions and discusses the many pressures experienced by families.

The other six chapters in the book are not directly linked to the discussion of the empiric data collected in the context of the European project or to the ethical or legal analysis of the complexity of predictive and prenatal testing that was made in this context. Chapter 5 by Yapijakis *et al.* presents data on predictive and prenatal testing for HD in five European countries: Greece, Germany, Austria, Switzerland and Denmark. Chapter 7 by Geraedts and Liebaers starts with an informative part on the PGD procedure before discussing the different types of PGD for HD. Thereafter, they discuss the experiences in Maastricht and Brussels in a more detailed way and also refer to the experience of other centres in the world. In Chapter 8 de Die and Heurckmans give case presentations concerning the use of PGD and give a clear picture of the meaning that it has for a number of families. Because of the need to guarantee anonymity a number of details have been changed but the key aspects of the families' experience have been fully respected. Whereas most of the other chapters in the book focus mainly on HD (with or without an extension to other neurogenetic disease), Chapter 11 by Dürr and Feingold starts with the presentation of the clinical and molecular features of the autosomal dominant hereditary ataxias and presents data on the demand for predictive and prenatal testing for this group of diseases. In Chapter 12 Craufurd discusses the counselling aspects of prenatal testing for late-onset neurogenetic diseases, paying particular attention to the implications for the situation of the existing and subsequent children and to the sex of the at-risk parent. Whereas all of the previous chapters focused mainly, but not exclusively, on Europe, Chapter 13 by Nance deals with predictive and prenatal testing for neurogenetic late-onset diseases in North America. In chapter 14 Harper gives some personal comments on the other chapters and on the radical changes that the field will probably see in the future.

References

Adam, S., Wiggins, S., Whyte, P., et al (1993) Five year study of prenatal testing for Huntington's disease: demand, attitudes and psychological assessment. *J. Med. Genet.* **30:** 549–556.

Craufurd, D., Dodge, A., Kerzin-Storrar, L. and Harris, R. (1989) Uptake of presymptomatic predictive testing for Huntington's disease (letter). *Lancet* **2:** 603–605.

Decruyenaere, M., Evers-Kiebooms, G., Boogaerts, A., Cassiman, J.J., Cloostermans, T., Demyttenaere, K., Dom, R., Fryns, J.-P. and Van den Berghe, H. (1997) Non participation in predictive testing for Huntington's disease: individual decision making, personality and avoidment behavior in the family. *Eur. J. Hum. Genet.* **5:** 351–363.

Evers-Kiebooms, G. (1997) Recent evolutions in prenatal testing for Huntington's disease. Presentation during the 17th International Meeting of the World Federation of Neurology Research Group on Huntington's Disease, Sydney, August.

Evers-Kiebooms, G. and Decruyenaere, M. (1998) Predictive testing for Huntington's disease: a challenge for persons at risk and for professionals. *Patient Educ. Counsel.* **35:** 15–26.

Evers-Kiebooms, G., Fryns, J.P., Demyttenaere, K., Decruyenaere, M., Boogaerts, A., Cloostermans, T., Cassiman, J.-J., Dom, R. and Van den Berghe, H. (1996) Predictive and preimplantation genetic testing for Huntington's disease and other late-onset dominant disorders: not in conflict but complementary (letter). *Clin. Genet.* **50:** 275–276.

Evers-Kiebooms, G., Welkenhuysen, M., Claes, E., Decruyenaere, M. and Denayer, L. (2000) The psychological complexity of predictive testing for late onset neurogenetic diseases and hereditary cancers. *Soc. Sci. Med.* **51:** 831–841.

Harper, P. (1996) *Huntington's Disease.* Saunders, London.

Harper, P. and Clarke, A. (1997) *Genetics, Society and Clinical Practice.* BIOS Scientific Publishers, Oxford.

Harper, P., Lim, C. and Craufurd, D. (2000) Ten years of presymptomatic testing for Huntington's disease: the experience of the U.K. Huntington's Disease Prediction Consortium. *J. Med. Genet.* **37:** 567–571.

Hayden, M.R. (2001) Predictive testing for Huntington Disease – 15 years later. Presentation during the International Congress of Human Genetics in Vienna, 15 May.

Hayden, M.R., Bloch, M. and Wiggins, S. (1995) Psychological effects of predictive testing for Huntington's disease. *Behav. Neurol. Mov. Disord.* **65:** 201–210.

Huntington's Disease Collaborative Research Group (1993) A novel gene containing a trinucleotide repeat that is expanded and unstable on Huntington's disease chromosomes. *Cell* **72:** 971–983.

International Huntington Association and World Federation of Neurology (1994) Guidelines for the molecular genetics predictive test in Huntington's disease. *Neurology* **44:** 1533–1536.

Quaid, K.A. and Morris, M. (1993) Reluctance to undergo predictive testing: the case of Huntington disease. *Am. J. Med.* **45:** 41–45.

Rowland, L.P. and Shneider, N.A. (2001) Amyotrophic lateral sclerosis. *N. Engl. J. Med.* **344:** 1688–1700.

Schulman, J.D., Black, S.H., Handyside, A. and Nance, W.E. (1996) Preimplantation genetic testing for Huntington's disease and certain other dominantly inherited disorders. *Clin. Genet.* **49:** 57–58.

ipt.

Tibben, A., Niermeijer, M.F., Roos, R.C., Vegter-van der Vlis, M., Frets, P.G., van Ommen, G.J., van de Kamp, J.J. and Verhage, F. (1992) Understanding the low uptake of presymptomatic DNA-testing for Huntington's disease (letter). *Lancet* **340:** 1416.

Tolmie, J.L., Davidson, H.R., May, H.M., McIntosh, K., Paterson, J.S. and Smith, B. (1995) The prenatal exclusion test for Huntington's disease: experience in the west of Scotland, 1986–1993. *J. Med. Genet.* **32:** 97–101.

Tyler, A., Ball, D. and Craufurd, D. (1992) Presymptomatic testing for Huntington's disease in the United Kingdom. *Br. Med. J.* **304:** 1593–1596.

Tyler, A., Quarrell, O., Lazarou, L.P., Meredith, A.L. and Harper, P.S. (1990) Exclusion testing in pregnancy for Huntington's disease. *J. Med. Genet.* **27:** 488–495.

Van der Steenstraten, I., Tibben, A., Roos, R.A., Van de Kamp, J.J. and Niermeijer, M.F. (1994) Predictive testing for Huntington disease: nonparticipants compared with participants in the Dutch program. *Am. J. Hum. Genet.* **55:** 618–625.

2

Case histories of prenatal testing for Huntington's disease

Gioia Jacopini, Marleen Decruyenaere, Ruth Harper and Sheila A. Simpson

1. Introduction

The increased availability of prenatal testing offers women prenatal results about many disorders even though treatment or cure is impossible for almost all of them. Yet, women usually ask for prenatal testing on the assumption that they must make every possible effort to foster the health of their children. All the more reason if they feel directly responsible because they are personally at risk for a genetic disease. Prenatal diagnosis, however, presents a wide range of decisions and challenges as is evident in the following case histories concerning requests for prenatal diagnosis in Huntington's disease (HD). In addition, these cases highlight some of the difficult problems that couples at risk for HD face if they want to have children.

The five cases are from European countries and the four genetic centres in which these couples were seen provided them with genetic counselling and additional psychological support. The procedures for prenatal testing in each centre are comparable (Chapter 4) and in all cases the prospective parent at risk was the mother.

Notwithstanding these similarities, these case histories are highly individual stories: each is important in itself, each experience is useful in gaining some knowledge that can be of help to others. The authors have tried to unravel the conscious, as well as unconscious, components of these five couples' decision-making processes. Seizing the differences helps to better understand the complexity of living under the shadow of a high genetic risk. The real reasons underlying women's decisions to undergo prenatal testing require a better understanding, especially in those cases in which the woman and her fetus share the same condition of genetic risk. A genetic disease is not just a physical

Prenatal Testing for Late-Onset Neurogenetic Diseases, edited by G. Evers-Kiebooms, M. W. Zoeteweij and P. S. Harper
©2002 BIOS Scientific Publishers Ltd, Oxford

status of the body. It is also a social product as well as a main component of the at-risk individual's identity.

In order to respect the privacy and confidentiality of the families some details, irrelevant to the meaning of the stories, have been changed.

2. Prenatal genetic testing for Huntington's disease: a particular aspect of mother–child relationship

The availability of prenatal testing shapes the experiences of maternity and establishes 'responsible' behaviours. Even though no treatments are available for almost all the disorders that can be detected, women undergo prenatal testing in order to ensure their children's health.

Although presented as a reassuring routine, prenatal testing may, however, raise more concerns than it can answer, for instance, in those cases in which the woman and her fetus are both at risk for the same genetic disease.

The first case history reported here is of a woman at risk for HD who opted for the exclusion test in pregnancy. Her intention to terminate the pregnancy in case of a 50% risk fetus, expressed before the test, was reversed after the communication of an unfavourable test result (status of the fetus equal to the status of the mother) and she decided to carry the pregnancy to term.

Now, 10 years after making that choice, she begins to perceive herself as symptomatic. In this situation, the onset of the disease in the mother heralds that her child too will be affected. This experience shows that the most commonly given reason for prenatal testing, such as preventing the birth of affected individuals, may raise conflicts in those cases in which the mother herself is at risk and is trying to assert the value of her own life. In fact, the choice this woman made of continuing with the pregnancy is easier to understand in the context of her life, the life of a person at 50% risk for HD who felt that the decision to abort a 50% risk fetus would have had the unmistakable meaning of a self-devaluation.

This case history also underlines that the pregnant woman has a very complex relationship with the fetus that is both part of her body and a separate identity.

One of the most relevant aspects of prenatal testing in situations of genetic risk is that it involves the mother–child relationship and we need to achieve a broader understanding of what it means to be a mother in such difficult conditions.

2.1 Mrs O

Mrs O and her husband came to our genetic centre for the first time 10 years ago. At presentation the pregnancy was already initiated. The prospective parent at risk was the mother, a 35-year-old woman. The affected parent was her father. He was very irritable, with frequent outbursts for which he afterwards used to express deep regret to his wife and his only daughter, Mrs O. This difficult, but very much loved, father committed suicide at 59 years. He had two brothers and one sister and all of them showed the disease. One brother's wife committed suicide and her two sons both became affected and died in their mid–30s. All the family had such a hard experience of the disease that for all her life Mrs O's mother had been watching her daughter, scared of the possible beginning of symptoms.

Mrs O and her husband already had a 4-year-old child and no prenatal diagnosis had been performed during the first pregnancy. 'We had him in a period of optimism', she explained.

Mrs O reported that when the second, unplanned pregnancy had begun, she felt 'a duty' to know about the future child. Given the tragic effects of the disease on her family, she did not want to know about herself because she considered it would be very difficult, even impossible, to live with a bad result. Prenatal exclusion testing was offered. During the counselling session, prenatal exclusion testing was explained in detail to the couple and all the implications of carrying the pregnancy to term after a possible unfavourable prenatal test result were illustrated. Mrs O understood all the explanations on a rational level and expressed the intention to terminate the pregnancy in case of non-exclusion. Her internal attitude was that she expected a favourable prenatal test result because, as she said: 'I deserve a little bit of luck after so many years misfortune!'.

The husband was more in favour of also having the second pregnancy without any prenatal diagnosis but he readily accepted her opposing decision saying that she would have got her own way in any case. The test was performed and gave an unfavourable result, a 50% risk fetus. The unfavourable prenatal test result shattered her expectations of 'compensation' from destiny and at first she was sad and resentful. A couple of days later the previously stated intention to terminate the pregnancy in case of a 50% risk fetus was reversed and Mrs O informed us that she had decided to carry the pregnancy to term. She said that she had been considering her life and the life of her future child and her conclusion was: 'I cannot terminate the pregnancy of a baby who is like me. I feel it would mean that I consider my life as not worth living. You know, I feel as if I would abort myself'.

Her husband's attitude was that of leaving the final decision to her protecting himself behind the screen that: 'It's up to the woman deciding about the pregnancy'.

Now, 10 years after that first contact, Mrs O called our genetic centre asking for presymptomatic testing. She was very anxious and said: 'I see my mother looking at my face . . . no, it would be better to say that she avoids looking at my face and I am sure this means that she thinks I am symptomatic. I must know'.

She came with her husband and we explored all the pros and cons of knowing, including the violation of her child's right to not know if she turned out to be a carrier. In the end she decided not to undergo the presymptomatic genetic testing but rather to wait and see what happened and her husband agreed with her. Mrs O explained her choice saying that her mother was old and weak after recent cancer surgery and that in the case of an unfavourable predictive test result she would never be able to hide the truth from her mother: 'Our communication has always been almost telepathic. She would immediately know the truth'.

In subsequent counselling sessions we have also been exploring her feelings about the implications for her second child, who is now 10 years old, of her eventually becoming symptomatic. Mrs O said: 'If I have got the disease I will never tell him that he is like me. In some way, you know, I start thinking he really is not like me because he is not necessarily going to have my same destiny. He is so young, I mean, and even though my mother is right, if I am sick now, I am 45 and this means that there are 35 years before he develops the disease and I am sure. . . I hope. . . a cure will be available by that time'.

2.2 Comments

Pregnancy is usually described in terms of either the woman and her rights or the fetus and its rights. Terms and concepts such as choice, autonomy and rights, however, do not describe the essence of this pregnancy. In some way, these perspectives tend to oversimplify matters.

Women's experience of pregnancy is complex: as is evident in this case, the pregnant woman considers herself to be involved in a relationship with the fetus that is both part of the woman's body and a distinct entity. As we have seen, although during pregnancy Mrs O identified herself with the fetus and for this reason did not terminate the pregnancy of a 50% risk fetus (. . .I feel as if I would abort myself) now, under the growing fear of becoming symptomatic, she activates a defensive strategy and begins to consider her 10-year-old child as a distinct entity (. . .I start thinking he really is not like me. . .). Moreover, the woman and her fetus are not isolated: they have relationships with previous children, with a spouse, with other family members and the decisions the pregnant woman takes involve all these other relationships. In this case, family relationships had been deeply influenced by the disease: HD, suicide and tragic early deaths were so closely intertwined in Mrs O's life experience as to make unbearable for her even the idea of living with a bad personal predictive test result. She could live only in the hope of not being a carrier and moreover, she considered that she deserved this as compensation from destiny for having stolen her father, cousins, aunts and uncles, and also the happy adolescence she had a right to. She had her first child without any prenatal diagnosis 'in a period of optimism', as she said. In the second pregnancy, in contrast, she felt 'the duty to know'. However, this 'duty to know' was not in terms of a technological imperative: she had easily ignored every prenatal technology during the first pregnancy. For the second pregnancy 'optimism' was no longer sufficient, she needed to be reassured, to have tangible proof that destiny really was compensating her. When the unfavourable prenatal test result arrived, she reacted to the ill fortune by using her, and her fetus's, 50% chance of not being carriers as the basis for again building up her hopes and expectations of 'compensation' from destiny. Only in hope can she live.

Reproductive genetic testing raises complex issues. One of the reasons is that these tests implicate the mother–child relationship and one of the most complex aspects of this relationship, in the context of genetics and prenatal diagnosis of disease, is that it also includes the possibility that the mother feels that the best relationship she can have with the child is not to be a mother and to terminate the pregnancy.

The choice Mrs O made of carrying the pregnancy to term after the unfavourable prenatal test result may be difficult to understand unless we consider it in the context of the circumstances of her life where it makes a great deal of sense.

Prenatal diagnosis is a situation in which someone has to choose: it is the meaning of this choice in terms of the at-risk individual's personal/family life, in terms of the parent–child relationship that appears to be one of the main aspects in this matter. There is need for a broader and inclusive understanding of what it means to be a mother, of what parenting entails in conditions of risk for a severe genetic disease, such as HD: the choice this woman made during pregnancy is contextual, not abstract. So should our understanding be.

3. Prenatal genetic testing for Huntington's disease and the technological imperative: a case presentation

Some couples who consider having children following an unfavourable predictive test result feel a pressure to use prenatal diagnosis simply because the technology is available. This phenomenon is known as the 'technological imperative'. The technological imperative impedes couples from considering other possibilities, such as having no children or having children without medical intervention. The consequence may be repeated prenatal tests, with a lot of psychological suffering after successive terminations of pregnancy without reflection about the pathway chosen or about other possible pathways.

The case presentation illustrates a history of repeated prenatal tests. We present the reproductive decision-making process of a young woman who is carrier of the Huntington mutation and we try to unravel the role of the technological imperative in this process. The story underlines the importance of counselling before every pregnancy (and after each termination). Careful counselling should allow couples to obtain insight into their beliefs, motives and feelings so that free informed choices are facilitated.

3.1 Mrs K

Mrs K is the youngest girl in a family of four children. She has two older sisters and one younger brother. Her parents run a greengrocer's shop. Mrs K and her three siblings are at 50% risk for developing HD. The first motor symptoms in Mrs K's mother appeared in her early 40s. Mother became gradually more irritable, explosive and hypersensitive and memory, reasoning and planning deteriorated little by little. Mother neglected her children and was no longer able to organize the housekeeping. At that time, Mrs K was between 12 and 15 years old. She knew that her mother 'behaved herself in the same way as her grandmother and as her aunt did' and Mrs K was very anxious that she would become just like them when grown up. Mother was diagnosed as having HD about 2 years later. Some years thereafter, an admission into a psychiatric hospital was necessary.

Mrs K and her siblings took their high school education at a boarding school. During the weekend, the three girls took care of the housekeeping. Immediately after high school, Mrs K looked for a job. At the time of the predictive test, Mrs K was 25 years old, she worked at a flower shop and she felt happy in her job. Mrs K married John when she was 22 years old. She and her partner visited Mrs K's mother on a regular basis.

Three years after marriage, the young couple came to the genetic centre and asked for the predictive test. The major reason for the test request was getting rid of the uncertainty. Mrs K suffered a lot from being at risk. A second reason was their desire to have children who would not carry the Huntington mutation. Mrs K had a normal personality profile and good personal resources. She had an intermediate level of general anxiety, but a high level of HD-related anxiety during the counselling sessions. She was not depressed. Her most common coping styles were avoiding behaviour and seeking distraction and amusement to escape from negative thoughts. Mrs K's partner had a good ego-strength and was not anxious. He was an important support person for Mrs K, as was one of her sisters. No other family member or friend was informed about her predictive test request. Before the test, they had made arrangements for a trip immediately after the test result to set aside their grief and worry in the case of an unfavourable test result, and to celebrate in the case of a favourable result.

Mrs K received an unfavourable test result. Immediately after the test result, the couple went for a trip with friends, who were not informed about the predictive test and the test result.

About 1 month after the test, Mrs K had told her father about the unfavourable test result, as well as her two sisters, her brother and a good friend. At that moment, her HD-related anxiety was lower than in the pretest period. The couple seemed to cope well with the test result. However, they avoided talking or thinking about the test result and its implications and tried to escape from negative thoughts and feelings by travelling and other pleasure-seeking behaviour. During the counselling session, the desire to have a child was raised again and the possible options were discussed with the couple: having children without medical intervention, having children with prenatal diagnosis or *in vitro* fertilization (IVF) with a donor egg. It was very clear for Mrs K that she did not want to pass the mutation to her children and that she wanted genetic testing of the fetus during pregnancy. In-depth counselling revealed that Mrs K had a very strong desire to have a child, and that it was very important for her that this child did not carry the Huntington mutation. Her partner John conformed completely to Mrs K's wishes. Mrs K's strong desire to have a child that would not develop HD seemed, in part, to be a way of compensating for her own bad test result. Becoming a parent herself and the joy of motherhood might have comforting aspects for Mrs K and might help her to deny the test result. Mrs K avoided talking about the psychological burden for her child as a result of having a parent with HD in the future.

Some months later Mrs K was pregnant and underwent prenatal testing in our hospital. The fetus proved to be a carrier of the Huntington mutation and the pregnancy was terminated. During the counselling session, Mrs K said that she could not be happy with the pregnancy or be attached to the child until she knew that the fetus was free of the Huntington mutation.

Mrs K wanted to become pregnant again as soon as possible. About 7 months later, she was expecting again; prenatal testing again revealed an unfavourable test result and the pregnancy was terminated. Mrs K wanted to go on, and unfortunately, another pregnancy with an unfavourable predictive test result and pregnancy termination followed. Mrs K and her partner had a lot of sorrow about the successive bad results, but did not consider the option of having no children. During one of the counselling sessions, Mrs K stated that her sister, who had a 50% risk status, was pregnant at that moment and did not want to have prenatal testing. Mrs K's sister's reason for not wanting prenatal testing was the belief that a cure would be found before the child developed HD. The possibility of having a baby without medical intervention was again discussed with Mrs K, however, she did not want to consider that option: she was afraid that having a child who was possibly a mutation carrier would confront her with unbearable feelings of guilt and regret in the future. It was difficult for Mrs K to understand that a couple could decide to have a child without the certainty that this child would be free of HD. At that time, Mrs K and John asked for information about preimplantation genetic diagnosis (PGD), which had become available during the past year. However, at that moment, they hesitated because of the low success rate and the physical and psychological burden of this procedure.

After each termination, Mrs K had sick leave of some days. The couple regularly made a trip, alone or with friends, to rest and relax. Mrs K's partner was her prop and stay during this strenuous period. The couple was also supported by Mrs K and John's family, some good friends and by hospital staff members. Mrs K and John decided to make a final attempt by prenatal testing. If the next pregnancy had to be terminated again, they intended to proceed with PGD. Again, they had bad luck and had a fourth pregnancy terminated.

The couple proceeded with PGD. During the counselling session after the first unsuccessful implantation trial, Mrs K expressed the feeling that the grief and disappointment after an unsuccessful cycle was smaller than after an unfavourable prenatal test. After three unsuccessful trials, Mrs K was eventually pregnant with a child who was a non-carrier of the Huntington mutation. In the 11th week of this pregnancy, a prenatal test was performed for a last control of the non-carrier status of the fetus. The pregnancy evolved without difficulties. And in the spring, 4 years after Mrs K's predictive test result, a healthy boy was born.

A recent home visit showed that the young family is very happy. Mrs K and John, who is a florist, have started their own flower shop. They enjoy the growth of their son and the little joys of life. They try to live in the present and to avoid thinking of the future. However, they have made practical and financial arrangements to prepare for Mrs K's future disease. John and Mrs K have decided to have no further children. The visits to Mrs K's mother, who has mentally deteriorated now, are the most difficult moments in Mrs K's life.

3.2 Comments

It is clear that an unfavourable predictive test result confronts young couples of reproductive age with complex and burdensome decisions concerning family planning. All kinds of factors may play a role in this decision-making process: the strength of the desire to have children, personal family history, moral values, expectations regarding future treatment or cure and availability of pre-natal technology. The availability of prenatal technology generally does not simplify reproductive decision-making. Some couples '. . . felt that the avail-ability of the (prenatal) test impelled them to use it in the first pregnancy. Then, they could only justify the initial use of prenatal testing if they continued to use the same technology in future pregnancies.' (Adam *et al.*, 1993). This illustrates that some couples feel a pressure to use prenatal diagnosis because the tech-nology is available. This 'technological imperative' deters couples from consid-ering other possibilities, such as having no children or having children without medical intervention. The consequence may be repeated prenatal tests, without reflection about the pathway chosen or about other possible pathways.

The question may arise as to whether Mrs K and John were victims of the 'technological imperative' to use prenatal testing or PGD. In other words, did they feel a pressure to undergo these medical interventions only because the technology was available? Or did they have other (additional) reasons to continue with prenatal testing and PGD?

These questions are difficult to answer in a straightforward manner. The decision process to undergo prenatal testing followed by selective abortion is very complex and contains conscious, as well as unconscious, components. The most obvious reason to use prenatal testing is to prevent the birth of a child who is a carrier of the Huntington mutation. However, prospective parents are of course also influenced by several other conscious and unconscious arguments. The availability of medical technology does not automatically lead to its use, witness the low uptake of prenatal testing for HD (see Chapters 3 and 4).

It is our opinion that Mrs K's reproductive decisions were in the first place influenced by her strong desire to have a child that would not be at risk for HD. By having a baby that would not be at risk and that would not develop HD, she unconsciously tried to compensate for her own suffering from being at risk at a young age. Moreover, the relief and the peace of mind because this child would not be at risk for HD, had to counterbalance the grief and despair about her own future illness. Becoming a parent herself and the joy of motherhood might also have comforting aspects for Mrs K and might help her to deny her own unfavourable test result. A remarkable observation was that Mrs K completely denied the psychological burden for her child as a result of having a parent with HD in the future.

During the counselling before and after each pregnancy, other options for reproduction had been discussed with the couple; however, these were not acceptable to Mrs K. Her reaction contrasted with that of another couple who showed relief when they heard that the use of medical interventions for reproduction after an unfavourable predictive test result was not the only option. Although Mrs K and her partner considered the medical technology as an opportunity rather than a pressure, we cannot rule out the possibility that they unconsciously felt a pressure to continue to use this technology to justify their previous choices and to make up for the previous losses. During counselling, we had discussed with the couple that feelings or circumstances may have changed after each prenatal testing situation, and that careful consideration had to be made before deciding about the next pregnancy. However, it was undoubtedly very difficult for the couple to abandon their chosen pathway. The feeling that all the suffering would have been in vain if they stopped the medical interventions had grown exponentially after each failed pregnancy and might be unbearable for the couple. The idea that the communication of 'good news' would eventually compensate for all the previous effort and suffering may have forced the couple to go on with the prenatal testing and later on, with the PGD.

Another aspect playing a very important role in Mrs K's (continued) choice for medical technology was her anticipated regret and feelings of guilt should she have a child that might be at risk. Indeed, preventing feelings of regret regarding the choices one has made proved an important motivational factor in decision-making (Tijmstra, 1989). In the context of reproductive decisions and prenatal testing, this means that some individuals use prenatal testing because they fear future feelings of regret and guilt, if they do not try everything possible to have a 'healthy child'. These future feelings of guilt and regret may especially be induced when the child or others ask for justification about the parents' decision-making. In the case of Mrs K and John, it is clear the anticipated guilt and regret of their decision may also have played an important role in the decision to continue with prenatal testing. The same psychological mechanism had an influence in the later decision to proceed with PGD.

It is clear that the technological imperative was not the only mechanism that played a role in Mrs K's reproductive decision-making process. Her decisions were also a coping strategy to deal with her own history and future illness and to prevent the future burden of shame and guilt. Finally, we cannot rule out that Mrs K stuck to the same choices in each pregnancy for other reasons, including her feelings of imperfection as a wife and mother, i.e. feeling unable to have a healthy child.

4. An example of a prenatal request for Huntington's disease masking underlying marital conflict

The following case report illustrates that requests for prenatal testing may mask deeper issues within the individual or relationship and that these may only become apparent within the counselling framework.

4.1 Miss A

Miss A first presented to the genetics service aged 26 years to discuss possible genetic testing for herself for HD. She was at 50% risk. She had recently become involved in a new relationship, her partner, 40 years old, having previously been married with three healthy children. She was aware of the many aspects of HD as her affected father had died 2 years previously and she had been involved in caring for him since her mother left the family home in the early stages of the illness. He had become affected aged 42 years.

The initial contact was precipitated by her new relationship and neither felt that it was an appropriate time to pursue presymptomatic testing. Within the consultation both expressed the feeling that their relationship was long-term, but that neither wished to have children.

There was initial follow-up and then no contact until 5 years later when Miss A contacted the department to request an appointment as she was now 10 weeks pregnant. During the initial telephone contact she expressed satisfaction with the pregnancy and a desire to discuss possible options for prenatal testing.

Miss A and her partner both attended the consultation. Miss A again initially expressed satisfaction with what was described as an unplanned pregnancy. However, her partner indicated his opposition to the pregnancy. He had children from a previous marriage and felt both that he did not wish to father any more children nor could they afford it in view of his pre-existing financial commitments. He had understood that she had also rejected the possibility of children because of the risk of HD.

As the interview progressed it was clear that the issue of children had been an unresolved area of disagreement from the start of their relationship and that both had underestimated the depth of the other's feelings. During the consultation both attempted to recruit the counsellors to their position and it was clear that they had been unable to resolve the issues before attending. Possible options for prenatal testing were discussed which Miss A wished to explore in detail. The interview terminated with her decision to consider direct testing of the pregnancy; her partner did not support the decision. Arrangements were made for them to be seen again but prior to that Miss A telephoned the department to say that she had undergone a termination of the pregnancy. She had felt that to continue with it would have jeopardized her relationship with her partner and she was not prepared to attempt to raise a child as a single parent.

Subsequent follow-up over the next 6 months revealed further issues within the relationship and they parted after a further 3 months.

4.2 Comments

The case illustrates that although the initial contact was for advice about prenatal testing in an apparently stable relationship, at consultation it was evident that this was being used as a vehicle to attempt to resolve a longstanding dispute within the relationship and was indicative of deeper dysfunction. The ultimate outcome of the pregnancy was neither dependent on nor decided by factors related to HD.

5. Two women at risk of Huntington's disease: two families with different decisions

Two cases concerning multiple requests for prenatal diagnosis in HD are given. Both women chose the same path as they made their choices about their pregnancies but ultimately made different choices for themselves.

5.1 Mrs AB

Mrs AB was 30 years old at presentation. She and her husband had no children, although she was in her second marriage. She is part of a sibship of four, and was aware that there was a history of HD in the family. Her paternal grandmother had been affected. At the time of presentation, her father had not been diagnosed with HD, but there were family concerns that he was exhibiting features of the disease. Initially, this woman sought presymptomatic predictive testing, and efforts were made to collect relevant samples from the rest of the family so that linkage analysis could be undertaken. It emerged that her father's sister had just had the diagnosis made, and the issue was clearly a sensitive one for the family.

Mrs AB's commitment to testing for herself meant that she took her father and mother to see the geneticist for sample collection for the family study, and it was at this appointment that the diagnosis was made formally in her father. Mrs AB's mother and father were aware that he had problems, and expected an opinion of his status. It was their first contact with a doctor to discuss his family history of HD and his own possible diagnosis. This was an extraordinarily difficult appointment for Mrs AB who felt that her own desire for information had resulted in her parents having to confront the disease in her father. In addition, the 50% risk to Mrs AB and her three siblings was confirmed.

Mrs AB became pregnant. She had joined the presymptomatic predictive testing programme and had discussions about the implications of the test for herself and her partner, and time for informed reflection. She decided that she would not undergo predictive testing herself, but rather have exclusion testing in her pregnancy. The result was unfavourable and the pregnancy was terminated. In the following 6 years, Mrs AB was pregnant five times, only the third pregnancy was continued as it was a favourable result.

The fifth and last pregnancy took place after the mutation causing HD had been described. Mrs AB decided that she still did not wish to ascertain her status, and accordingly exclusion testing was again requested. After this fifth pregnancy, the couple decided that their family was complete. The couple were very sure about their approach to dealing with the risk of HD to their children, but nonetheless did not feel able to continue with a further pregnancy.

This case illustrates the concerns of at-risk individuals about ascertaining their own status, but nonetheless wishing not to transmit the at-risk status to any child they might have. Mrs AB was in her second marriage, and keen not to have this relationship threatened in any way. Her husband was very supportive of all her decisions, but she was very aware that an unfavourable predictive test result could prejudice their relationship.

Their wish to have children was strong, but not at the cost of transmission of the disease, and not at the cost of endangering their marriage and their time together.

A further issue for this woman was the definition of the status of her father. She felt that her mother required support and that her father required medical care which he was not receiving as he had no diagnosis. She was also concerned that her siblings realize their risk. She was anxious that signs of the disease were evident in two other family members. None of Mrs AB's siblings confronted their fears about the disease before she took her father to the clinic, and she felt a considerable responsibility for producing such information.

5.2 Comments

At her last review Mrs AB has no regrets about her past decisions, and remains sure that she does not wish presymptomatic predictive testing.

The advent of mutation testing did not alter Mrs AB's decision about need to remove 'the' predictive testing for her or the mode of testing of her pregnancies. The counsellor felt it important that her own at-risk status was preserved and that no information should be produced which would prejudice this.

5.3 Mrs CD

Mrs CD was aged 25 years at presentation. The history of HD was well known in the family, but never discussed. Mrs CD's father was at 50% risk, but had not, to Mrs CD's knowledge, had predictive testing. An aunt was affected, and was a constant presence during Mrs CD's childhood. A source of distress to her was the lack of discussion about the signs of the disease in this person, and the fear which she felt when she met this woman. She felt that her aunt had not been treated with respect, and had regrets about this.

Mrs CD was very close to her parents and her two siblings, but was not able to share her fears about the disease with them. In particular, she did not feel that she could approach her father about his risk, as he might then feel that he had to undergo predictive testing, which might produce unfavourable information for herself and her siblings.

She had complete confidence in the support and loyalty of her husband, but felt that she could not cope with an unfavourable presymptomatic predictive test result herself, especially as this would indicate her father's status, and increase the risk to her siblings.

Mrs CD's experience of being at risk of HD had dominated her teenage years. She did not want to inflict this experience on any children she might have, and when she became pregnant she sought exclusion testing for the pregnancy. It is clear that in some instances, and in this family, fear of the unknown and misinformation, contribute to the anxiety of individuals at risk of HD.

Her need for complete confidentiality from her father meant that a blood sample from him could not be requested for the family study. She did confide in her mother, and her sample was obtained. The family was informative and Mrs CD subsequently investigated four pregnancies. Two of these pregnancies were found to be at high risk and were terminated. She kept her pregnancies secret until the favourable results were obtained, and did not discuss the two terminations with her family.

The mutation responsible for HD was described soon after her fourth pregnancy was terminated, and after an interval of several months, she made a request for predictive testing. Her husband was aware and supportive, but she did not tell her parents of this decision. The result was favourable, and she went on to have further pregnancies. She has not informed her parents about the termination of the other pregnancies, or that she has undergone predictive testing and received a favourable result. To do this would cause her father distress, as he has not had testing himself.

5.4 Comments

This case illustrates the importance of family loyalties and fear of information. Families share their genetic heritage, but often do not have equal knowledge of this heritage. Through fear of the consequences of sharing this information, and the need for their own privacy, many family members do not tell others about their fears, their investigations and their results.

This family still does not discuss HD, and Mrs CD continues to have concerns about her father's status. She is unaware if her siblings have sought advice. She has no regrets about her decisions in her pregnancies which she regards as the only possible route she could have followed at that time.

Mrs CD's experience of being at risk for HD meant that she would not have had children at all had she not been able to use exclusion testing. At that time in her marriage, both she and her husband wanted to have children, and the discovery of the Huntington mutation was still a long way in the future, with no certainty of being found. Her decision was based on having children or not, and once the gene was described, she could not negate her earlier feelings. She regrets the loss of her pregnancies, but not the decision to terminate them.

6. Conclusions

Pregnancy has different psychological meanings for prospective parents. The reasons underlying the desire to have children are usually complex and in most cases couples are not entirely conscious of all their motivations. When reproduction entails a risk for a severe genetic disorder the ambivalent elements can be intensified. The five case reports, although not representing the total experience of prenatal testing for HD, can help to understand how many different choices individuals at risk for, or carriers of, the Huntington's mutation can make in their reproductive decisional process. Individual's choices, in fact, are not only deeply influenced by the presence of the genetic risk in their life but also by the more general family style in managing the illness.

For individuals at risk for HD, to marry and have children means to have a 'normal' life and in some cases the desire of a compensative healthy child is so strong that they are ready to make very hard choices. As these stories highlight, in deciding whether to have the prenatal diagnosis they are influenced by many rational as well as irrational motives and the importance of counselling, pre- and post prenatal diagnosis, emerges with strong evidence: each case has been a challenge for the counsellor trying to help the counsellees obtain a better understanding of their reproductive motivations and to have an insight into the role played by possible hidden reasons in their choices.

From the stories it also emerges that nondirective counselling is an achievable goal: counsellors gave couples all the available information, furnished with them all the possible options and did their best to help them to explore the personal meaning of their ambivalent feelings and obtain a full understanding of all the factors influencing their decisional process.

The psychological aspects of abortion have been studied and it is well known that for many women it is a profound experience. Years afterwards they may still have painful feelings, even when aware that, under the same circumstances, they would probably decide to abort again.

In these case reports the emotional health of the women who underwent even repeated abortions does not seem to be undermined: they were able to make their choices with apparently little harm and few regrets.

In our opinion, one of the reasons for their looking back on their past decisions with no regrets is that the choice really rested with the couple and was the product of their ability to understand what was more appropriate for their specific needs and of the skill of the counsellor in providing psychological support, in respecting their decisions and in making them aware of, and prepared for, possible future problems.

References

Adam S, Wiggins S, Whyte P *et al*. (1993) Five year study of prenatal testing for Huntington's disease: demand, attitudes and psychological assessment. *J. Med. Genet.* **30:** 549–556.

Tijmstra, T. (1989) The imperative character of medical technology and the meaning of anticipated decision regret. *Int. J. Technol. Assess. Health Care* **5:** 207–213.

3

An overview of prenatal testing for Huntington's disease in six European countries

Moniek W. Zoeteweij, Kurt Nys, Peter S. Harper,
Sheila A. Simpson, Alexandra Dürr, Gioia Jacopini,
Christos Yapijakis and Gerry Evers-Kiebooms

1. Introduction

More than a century ago George Huntington (1850–1916) described a family with neurodegenerative symptoms in several generations and this disease became known as Huntington's disease (HD; Huntington, 1872). During the last two decades advances in molecular and genetic technology have generated new and far-reaching insights into the hereditary characteristics of the disease. Because the gene is known, each child of an affected parent has a 50% risk of having inherited the disease. The diagnosis of HD may have profound consequences for offspring: children at risk subsequently have to deal with the knowledge of having a severely ill parent with irreversible and progressive motor, neurological and personality impairments and they will be confronted with personal consequences for future and family planning (Harper, 1996).

In 1983, a major breakthrough revealed the location of the gene on chromosome 4p16.3 (Gusella *et al.*, 1983). Predictive testing became available by means of linkage analysis, identifying gene carriers or excluding carriership. For persons at risk for HD a new era began: predictive (presymptomatic) testing gave the option of acquiring information about one's genetic status before symptoms of the disease appear. The main disadvantages of linkage analysis were the possibility of receiving an uninformative test outcome and the need for family cooperation in blood sampling.

Prenatal Testing for Late-Onset Neurogenetic Diseases, edited by G. Evers-Kiebooms,
M. W. Zoeteweij and P. S. Harper
©2002 BIOS Scientific Publishers Ltd, Oxford

Linkage analyses gave 50% at-risk individuals the opportunity and hope of excluding carriership with high reliability. However, healthcare providers involved in genetic testing worried about the possible distressing and catastrophic consequences for those test applicants who turned out to be carriers. Predictive testing procedures were therefore implemented within a professional test protocol with multidisciplinary expertise.

New technological advances led to identification of the mutation in 1993 (Huntington Disease Collaborative Research Group, 1993). DNA testing then became an individual matter, meaning that each individual at risk could opt for testing without the need for family blood samples and with the certainty of receiving a highly reliable test outcome. Nevertheless, confirmation of the clinical diagnosis in at least one affected relative remains important. Although DNA testing became technically more straightforward, it also led to new ethical dilemmas. For instance, 25% at-risk individuals could apply for DNA testing against the wishes of their 50% at-risk parent. The disclosure of carriership in a 25% at-risk adult would establish that the parent is also a gene carrier and would alter the at-risk status of siblings (Simpson and Harding, 1993). This option raised the question of whose right carries most weight: the right of an adult child to know its genetic status or the right of a parent not to know.

Another dilemma concerns prospective parents at 50% risk who wish to exclude carriership in the fetus without revealing the genetic status of the parent, using the prenatal exclusion test. In the guidelines of the International Huntington Association and World Federation of Neurology Research Group on Huntington's Chorea (1994) it is stated that prenatal testing should be performed only if the parent's genetic status is known, except for prenatal exclusion testing. In this situation, the fetus is tested using chorion villus sampling and linkage analysis to determine whether the fetus has inherited a chromosome 4 from the affected grandparent. The outcome of the prenatal exclusion test does not change the risk of the prospective parent, whereas the fetus receives an (almost) zero risk or 50% risk. In the latter case, prospective parents usually decide to terminate the pregnancy.

During the earlier period of linkage testing, prenatal exclusion testing was the only option for couples with an uninformative predictive test result. After mutation detection became available, prenatal exclusion testing became a controversial instrument for at-risk couples who did not want to know the genetic status of the future parent but explicitly wanted to exclude carriership in their offspring. Non-exclusion of the gene implied that prospective parents consciously decide for a pregnancy termination with a 50% chance of aborting a non-affected fetus. For those parents at risk it is important to realize that they may eventually discover that he or she is not a carrier implicating that a pregnancy termination after prenatal exclusion testing has been unnecessary.

Mutation detection revealed even more complexities: the so-called 'grey zone' was discovered, i.e. individuals with intermediate alleles (27–35 CAG repeats) received a reduced (but not zero) risk that transmission might result in HD in their offspring (Kelly et al., 1999). It was assumed that couples with an intermediate allele might have difficulty in coping with family planning decisions. Furthermore, with mutation detection the accuracy of earlier results by linkage analyses could be retested on request and these procedures revealed some risk reversals with far-reaching consequences (Almqvist *et al.*, 1997).

The new advances in genetic technology also had major implications for genetic counselling as a discipline. Genetic counsellors had to deal with simplified technology and a more widespread acceptance of the predictive test, but also had to explain and discuss the more complex implications of the test for applicants and their families. For genetic counsellors and other professionals involved in the process of genetic testing technological progress implicated expert skills in communicating complex information.

Since the beginning, predictive testing has usually been offered at qualified genetic centres within the framework of a standardized protocol including genetic counselling and psychological support before and after test disclosure. After receiving predictive test results gene carriers may experience a short period of shock, anxiety, depression, worry and/or guilt followed by minor distress over the next 2 years with sometimes minimization of carriership (Bloch *et al.*, 1992; Codori and Brandt, 1994; Evers-Kiebooms *et al.*, 2000; Horowitz *et al.*, 2001; Lawson *et al.*, 1996; Tibben *et al.*, 1994). High-risk persons also reported relief from uncertainty about their genetic status. Very few catastrophic events, i.e. suicide attempts or psychiatric hospitalization, were reported in the first years after testing (Almqvist *et al.*, 1999) indicating that test applicants may be self-selected individuals who believe themselves to be better prepared to cope with unfavourable test results (Codori *et al.*, 1994). Contrary to expectations, in some persons with decreased risk relief was absent and numbed emotions and survivor guilt were found (Bloch *et al.*, 1992; Huggins *et al.*, 1992; Tibben *et al.*, 1994). These individuals may have overestimated the positive consequences of a decreased risk or may have made irreversible decisions based on the assumption that they would develop HD in the future. In the long-term some non-carriers still experience difficulties in planning a future without the perspective of having HD. The risk of HD may have influenced their personality development, hampering new self-definitions and engagements in relationships (Tibben *et al.*, 1997; Williams *et al.*, 2000). Bearing this in mind we may assume that a decreased risk may facilitate the decision to start a family, whereas this may also be restrained by difficulties with coping with a favourable test result. Although a considerable number of at-risk individuals applied for predictive testing because of family planning, the follow-up studies to date have not focused on the intentions and actual decision-making in reproduction after test disclosure.

This chapter will highlight the consequences of the accumulation of technological advances in HD leading to several technical options in prenatal testing.

2. Prenatal diagnosis as a reproductive choice of Huntington's disease family members

Identification of the gene has made it possible to offer predictive testing and prenatal diagnosis. Before the availability of prenatal testing future parents could refrain from procreation or accept the risk and decide to start a pregnancy with the uncertainty of transmitting the gene.

Because gene identification and mutation detection is possible, several options are technically available for individuals at risk regarding decision making in family planning: i.e. having a family without prenatal testing, refraining from having a family, prenatal diagnosis, prenatal exclusion testing, prenatal mutation testing without testing the parent first, preimplantation genetic diagnosis (PGD), donor sperm insemination/egg donation or adoption. Decision-making in reproduction is known to be an individual and complex process characterized by rational as well as irrational and unconscious motives (Frets *et al.*, 1990). Consequently, it is difficult to delineate the motives for deciding for prenatal diagnosis or one of the other options. It is inevitable that there are consequences for children despite the options in reproductive decision-making: e.g. even after prenatal exclusion of the gene the child will subsequently experience the impact of having a parent at risk for HD. Other concerns about possible negative consequences of prenatal diagnosis have been expressed, e.g. the so-called technological imperative referring to the strong social pressure to exclude carriership and the discrimination of parents who intentionally refrain from prenatal diagnosis. Another drawback in prenatal diagnosis was the expected severe distress of terminating a desired pregnancy.

Earlier surveys indicated that 30–80% of the individuals at risk intended to use prenatal diagnosis if available (Mastromauro *et al.*, 1987; Tyler *et al.*, 1990), but the actual uptake appears to be much lower (Adam *et al.*, 1993; Simpson and Harper, 2001). Results have indicated that the majority of individuals at risk declined prenatal testing because they felt that they could not terminate a pregnancy or because of the hope that a cure for HD would be found in time for their children.

In a pilot study about the attitudes of pregnant women with a high risk for HD it was observed that individuals were inclined to exclude carriership in their offspring. They started the process of decision-making for prenatal testing even before the predictive test of the parent was performed (Zoeteweij *et al.*, 1997). Applicants for prenatal diagnosis showed a tendency to minimize past experiences with their affected parent indicating that they avoided the negative consequences for their future children. Some high-risk individuals also advocated the potential support of future children for the non-HD parent after the decease of the parent at risk.

The actual uptake for pregnancy termination appears to be lower than applicants originally stated. Tolmie *et al.* (1995) described that of nine high-risk pregnancies three were continued despite the earlier expressed intention to terminate the pregnancy if the result indicated a high risk. One year after the predictive test result, Decruyenaere *et al.* (1996) found that one-third of carriers opted for prenatal testing, whereas one-third refrained from having children and one-third was undecided. Maat-Kievit *et al.* (1999) estimated the actual uptake for prenatal testing in The Netherlands as follows: at least 2% of individuals at 50% risk and 11% of the tested carriers applied for prenatal testing. In the UK, research has indicated that only a minority of those at risk for HD had chosen prenatal testing between 1994 and 1998 (Simpson and Harper, 2001).

To date, more information is needed about the actual uptake for prenatal diagnosis to understand more about the decisions of high-risk individuals regarding family planning. In clinical genetic centres there is sometimes the experience of few couples applying for prenatal diagnosis, little is known about those who hesitate or make other choices.

To gain more insight into the actual uptake of prenatal diagnosis for HD and into the psychological, legal and ethical implications, a European collaborative and multidisciplinary study was started in March 1998, including nine partners from six European countries who specialized in genetics, psychology, law and ethics, and including a representative from HD lay organizations. The aims of the European project have been thoroughly presented by Evers-Kiebooms (see Chapter 1). In Evers-Kiebooms *et al.* (submitted) a selection of the results of the European project about reproductive decision-making following predictive testing and uptake for prenatal testing in a group of mutation carriers is discussed.

This chapter focuses on the first aim of the collaborative study, i.e. creating a detailed picture of prenatal testing for HD in six European genetic centres with special focus on the type of the test (full prenatal testing, prenatal exclusion testing, guided exclusion testing). Other goals of the study are elaborated in later chapters.

The following sections present an overview of prenatal testing in the six participating countries. In particular, the following topics are addressed:

(i)   the sociodemographic characteristics of prospective parents at risk for HD and applying for prenatal testing;

(ii) the genetic status of prospective parents at risk for HD in relation to the type of prenatal test (full prenatal testing, exclusion, guided exclusion);

(iii) a detailed picture of repeated prenatal testing, i.e. couples at risk who had more than one prenatal test.

3. Study methods

In 1998, seven genetic centres from six European countries (Center for Human Genetics, Leuven, Belgium; Institute of Medical Genetics, Cardiff, UK; Dept of Human and Clinical Genetics, Leiden, The Netherlands; Département de génétique, cytogénétique et embryologie, Paris, France; Instituto di Psicologia, Rome, Italy; Dept of Neurology, Athens, Greece; Clinical Genetics, Aberdeen, UK) agreed to participate in a European collaborative study and began data collection about individual prenatal tests for HD. The data were gathered retrospectively from the start of the testing programme until 1999 in each centre (centre-level data) and it was also agreed to make an effort to collect data from 1993 to 1998 for each country (country-level data).

In Leuven, a questionnaire was composed including questions about the date of the predictive test, prospective mother or father belonging to the HD family, the genetic status of the prospective parent, the rank of the pregnancy, infor-mation about previous children and pregnancies, type and result of the prenatal test in the actual pregnancy and sociodemographic characteristics of the prospective parents (age, marital status and education). The type of prenatal test was categorized as: full prenatal test (linkage analysis or mutation analysis), prenatal exclusion test (linkage analysis to exclude carriership in the fetus and without changing the at-risk status of the prospective parent) and guided exclusion (including two steps: exclusion test followed by mutation analysis, only if the result of the exclusion test indicated a 50% risk for the fetus).

Data were retrieved from the medical files in the genetic centres, were anonymized and were sent to the coordinating centre of Leuven where the data were analysed. Descriptive statistics were used to summarize the data.

4. Results

Here the centre-level data are described in full, together with the country-level data. In some respects, the country-level data appeared incomplete and we therefore chose to leave out some of these data.

4.1 Sociodemographic characteristics of the prospective parents

In the six countries involved in the study, 305 prenatal tests were reported between 1993 and 1998.

Table 1 shows the number of reported prenatal tests per country with the highest numbers in the UK ($N = 157$) and The Netherlands ($N = 90$) and relatively low numbers in France ($N = 7$) and Greece ($N = 2$). Table 1 also shows the numbers of prenatal tests per centre (in total 202 prenatal tests). The different periods of data collection should be kept in mind: 1993–1998 for the country-level data and 1989–1999 for the centre-level data.

Table 1. Number of reported prenatal tests for Huntington's disease per country (1993–1998) ($N = 305$) and per centre (1988–1999) ($N = 202$)

Country level		Centre level		
	Number of tests		Number of tests	First test in
Belgium	30	Leuven	32	1988
Netherlands	90	Leiden*	124	1989
UK	157	Cardiff	11	1993
		Aberdeen	19	1989
France	7	Paris	7	1996
Italy	19	Rome	6	1990
Greece	2	Athens*	3	1991
Total	305		202	

*The number of prenatal tests in Leiden, The Netherlands, includes all prenatal tests in The Netherlands, because all DNA analyses for Huntington's disease are carried out in Leiden. The same is true for Athens, Greece.

Until 1994, Leiden was the only centre in The Netherlands performing predictive and prenatal testing for HD, partly explaining the relatively high numbers in Leiden compared with other centres. After 1994, the Leiden data still represent the data for The Netherlands, as the laboratory of human genetics in Leiden is the only centre performing DNA analysis for HD. Genetic counselling procedures have been decentralized since 1994 and are offered in seven clinical genetics centres in The Netherlands. Of the 124 prenatal tests carried out in The Netherlands, 90 received genetic counselling at the Department of Clinical Genetics in Leiden and 34 in one of the other centres. In Greece the centre in Athens performs all testing for HD.

Leuven reported that the first prenatal test was performed in 1988, Leiden and Aberdeen followed in 1989 and the other four centres reported their first prenatal test between 1990 and 1996.

The numbers of prenatal tests per year are shown in *Fig. 1*, indicating an increase in 1994 and stabilization with around 65 tests per year from 1996 to 1998.

Sociodemographic data about the prenatal test applicants were gathered for each prenatal test. Because some couples were involved in successive prenatal tests, it should be noted that sociodemographic data about the same person are included more than once. In addition, sociodemographic data are described for the data set with exclusively first prenatal tests (Section 4.3).

The mean age of prospective parents was 30.8 years for the country-level data (SD 4.27, range 17–41 years, $N = 167$; see *Table 2*). The mean age of the partners was 31.5 years (SD 3.75, range 19–42, $N = 133$) At the centre level the mean age of the individuals at risk was 30.5 years (SD 4.36, range 18–41), the mean age of the partners was 30.8 years (SD 4.17, range 19–45).

Forty-eight per cent of the prenatal tests were reported in married couples or couples within a stable relationship, in 48% of the tests the stability of the relationship was uncertain or unknown and in 4% the relationships were reported as unstable (country-level data). At the centre level, most tests (81%) were performed in persons within a stable relationship.

Retrospective data about the educational level of the couple at the time of the prenatal test were often missing and were left out of the presentation of results.

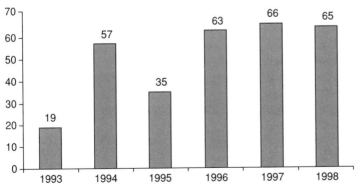

Figure 1. Number of reported prenatal tests for HD per year ($N = 305$, country-level data).

Table 2. Age of the prospective parent ($N = 305$, missing, 138)

Country	N	Mean	SD	Range
Belgium	29	30.2	3.80	24–40
Netherlands	88	30.9	4.07	18–40
UK	22	30.3	5.28	17–41
France	7	27.1	5.87	20–36
Italy	19	32.7	3.54	24–36
Greece	2	33.5	3.20	31–36
Total	167	30.8	4.27	17–41

In summary, the uptake for prenatal testing in the six countries in this European collaborative study appears to be low, with only 305 prenatal tests performed. Uptake was relatively high in the UK and The Netherlands compared with low numbers in France and Greece. The average age for applicants at risk was around 30 years and the majority was involved in a stable relationship.

4.2 Genetic characteristics of prospective parents and type of prenatal test

Data about the distribution between prospective mothers and fathers belonging to families with HD are given in *Table 3*. This shows that information at the country-level was missing in a substantial number of prenatal tests. In The Netherlands the majority of individuals were prospective mothers, whereas in the other five countries the distribution of mothers and fathers was almost equal.

When we look in more detail at the results for each participating centre Aberdeen and Leiden had more prospective mothers and Leuven and Cardiff more prospective fathers.

Table 3. Sex of prospective parents per country (1993–1998) ($N = 305$, missing, 114) and per centre (1988–1999) ($N = 202$, missing, 1)

	Country level			Centre level	
	Mother	Father		Mother	Father
Belgium	16	14	Leuven	8	24
Netherlands	54	36	Leiden	75	49
UK	20	23	Cardiff	3	7
			Aberdeen	15	4
France	4	3	Paris	4	3
Italy	8	11	Rome	3	3
Greece	1	1	Athens	2	1
Total	103	88	Total	110	91

The genetic status of the prospective parents is summarized in *Table 4*. Approximately half of the parents were asymptomatic gene carriers (51%), 42% were at risk, 6% were affected with HD and 1% were carriers of an intermediate allele. In the UK the number of affected prospective parents and the number of at-risk individuals were relatively high compared with the numbers in other countries. In Belgium, The Netherlands and France the majority of prospective parents were asymptomatic gene carriers. The centre-level data are in concordance with the above-mentioned: Cardiff, Aberdeen and Rome had more prenatal tests in couples at risk; in Leuven, Leiden and Paris more couples with an asymptomatic gene carrier applied for prenatal diagnosis.

As outlined above, prospective parents at risk have several options in reproductive decision-making. In our data, 198 tests (65%) were recorded as full prenatal tests with either linkage analysis or mutation testing. One hundred and five tests (35%) were prenatal exclusion tests.

The outcome of a prenatal exclusion test is either a decreased risk or 50% risk for the fetus, leaving the parent with 50% risk. In cases of a 50% risk outcome for the fetus parents may decide for or against pregnancy termination or decide for full testing (guided exclusion testing). In our series, Belgium, The Netherlands and France had more full prenatal tests (with the same tendencies in Leiden, Leuven, Paris and Athens). In the UK (Cardiff, Aberdeen) and Italy (Rome) the number of full prenatal tests almost equalled the number of exclusion tests (*Table 5*).

Table 4. Genetic status of the prospective parent per country (1993–1998) ($N = 305$, missing, 2) and per centre (1988–1999) ($N = 202$, missing, 0)

Country/centre	Affected	Asymptomatic carrier	Intermediate allele	At risk
Belgium	0	25	1	4
Leuven	0	30	0	2
The Netherlands	0	64	1	25
Leiden	0	73	1	50
UK	16	52	0	87
Cardiff	0	4	0	7
Aberdeen	1	1	0	17
France	0	5	0	2
Paris	0	5	0	2
Italy	0	8	1	10
Rome	0	0	0	6
Greece	1	0	0	1
Athens	1	1	0	1
Total country level	17	154	3	129
Total centre level	2	114	1	85

Table 5. Type of prenatal test per country (1993–1998) ($N = 305$) and per centre (1988–1999) ($N = 202$)

	Country level			Centre level	
	Full*	Exclusion†		Full*	Exclusion†
Belgium	27	3	Leuven	31	1
Netherlands	73	17	Leiden	83 (1)	41
UK	81	76	Cardiff	4	7
			Aberdeen	2	17
France	5	2	Paris	5	2
Italy	11 (2)	8	Rome	0	6
Greece	2	0	Athens	3	0
Total	199	106	Total	128	74

*Full, full prenatal test using linkage or mutation analysis; the guided exclusion test was used three times.
†Exclusion, prenatal exclusion test.

It was interesting to investigate the relation between the genetic status of the prospective parent and the type of prenatal test. Concerning the country-level data, the majority (81%) of prospective parents at risk had a prenatal exclusion test (*Table 6*). However, some of the at-risk individuals (19%) applied for full prenatal testing which is controversial because of the 25% chance of triple bad news, i.e. the fetus and the parent are both found to be carriers, followed by requested pregnancy termination. In the centre-level data the same trends were found. The high percentage of prenatal exclusion tests in this group is probably explained by the inclusion of prenatal tests performed before 1993, i.e. at that time for many families exclusion testing was the only option if they were to prevent transmission of the disease.

After disclosure of prenatal test results, 57% showed a decreased risk and 43% an increased risk. Almost the same results were found in the centre-level data. Eight pregnancies with an increased risk were continued (five in the UK, two in Italy and one in The Netherlands). Of these pregnancies six were tested using full prenatal testing and two using exclusion testing.

Table 6. The genetic status of the prospective parent in relation with the type of prenatal test per country (1993–1998) ($N = 305$) and per centre (1988–1999) ($N = 202$)

	Country level		Centre level	
Genetic status	Full*	Exclusion†	Full*	Exclusion†
Affected	17	0	2	0
Asymptomatic gene carrier	154	0	114	0
Intermediate allele	3	0	1	0
At risk	24 (2)	105	11 (1)	74
Total	198	105	128	74

*Full, full prenatal test using linkage or mutation analysis; the guided exclusion test was used three times.
†Exclusion, prenatal exclusion test.

In summary, the data indicate that more prospective mothers than prospective fathers belonging to a family with HD applied for prenatal testing. Especially in Aberdeen and Leiden, the majority of applicants were prospective mothers at risk; Leuven and Cardiff had more prospective fathers at risk. Furthermore, the majority of applicants were asymptomatic carriers in Leuven, Leiden and Paris, whereas we found more applicants at risk in Cardiff, Aberdeen and Rome, explaining a relatively high number of exclusion tests. In the UK a substantial number of affected applicants was reported. The majority of individuals at risk applied for exclusion testing. However, 24 couples at risk applied for full prenatal testing. With the exception of eight cases, all pregnancies with an increased risk were terminated.

4.3 Repeated prenatal testing

So far, we have focused on the prenatal test as the unit of observation. However, several couples had more than one pregnancy and they represent a special group of parents with repeated prenatal tests. Overall, 202 prenatal tests were performed in 129 couples in the seven participating centres; 41 couples had between 2 and 5 prenatal tests. Of the 129 couples, the mean age of the prospective parent at the time of the first prenatal test was 30.2 years (SD = 4.73). Seventy-three per cent of the first prenatal tests were requested by couples within a stable relationship, 5% of the relationships were qualified as unstable and 22% as uncertain or unknown.

Of the 129 couples with at least one prenatal test, 51% included a prospective mother belonging to the HD family and 49% a prospective father. In the 41 couples with more than one prenatal test, there was a slight tendency that the more prenatal tests the higher the chance of a prospective mother being involved (*Table 7*).

In the 129 couples with at least one prenatal test, 63% were full tests and 37% were exclusion tests. Fifty-two per cent of the prenatal test applicants were asymptomatic gene carriers, 46% included a person at risk for HD.

Table 7. Sex of the prospective parent in relation with repeated prenatal testing ($N = 41$, centre-level data)

Number of prenatal tests	Prospective mother ($N = 22$)	Prospective father ($N = 19$)
2	9	13
3	6	4
4	4	1
5	3	1

Table 8 shows the relation of the genetic status of the prospective parent at risk compared with the type of prenatal test: 11 of 59 persons were at risk and applied for full (linkage or mutation) prenatal testing.

Table 8. Status of the prospective parent in relation with the type of prenatal test ($N = 129$, centre-level data)

Genetic status	Full*	Exclusion†
Affected ($N = 2$)	2	0
Asymptomatic gene carrier ($N = 67$)	67	0
Intermediate allele ($N = 1$)	1	0
At risk ($N = 59$)	11 (1)	48
Total ($N = 129$)	81	48

*Full, full prenatal test using linkage or mutation analysis; the guided exclusion test was used once.
†Exclusion, prenatal exclusion test.

Table 9 shows a detailed picture of the test outcomes of couples with repeated prenatal tests. These results show that 88 of the 129 couples had one prenatal test. Twenty-five of the 129 couples proceeded with a second prenatal test after having had a favourable first prenatal test, whereas 15 couples with an unfavourable first prenatal test applied for a prenatal test in the next pregnancy.

Table 9. Prenatal test outcomes in couples with 1–5 prenatal tests ($N = 129$)
(U = unfavourable prenatal test result;
F = favourable prenatal test result)

Number of prenatal tests	Number of couples
1 ($N = 88$)	
U	56
F	32
2 ($N = 22$)	
F U	9
F F	9
U U	4
3 ($N = 10$)	
F F F	3
U U F	2
F U F	2
U F U	1
U F F	2
4 ($N = 5$)	
U U F F	1
F U U U	1
U F U F	1
F U U F	1
U U U U	1
5 ($N = 4$)	
F F U U U	1
U U F F F	1
U U U U U	2

The time interval between two consecutive prenatal tests in relation to the test result of the previous prenatal test is shown in *Table 10*. It is clear from these data that test applicants apply relatively quickly for a next prenatal test after receiving an unfavourable result in the previous pregnancy.

Seventeen couples applied for a next prenatal test within 6 months. Eleven of 27 couples waited more than 3 years after receiving a favourable result before they applied for prenatal testing in a new pregnancy, compared with 1 of 46 couples after receiving a previous unfavourable result.

In summary, approximately one-third of the applicants for prenatal testing had more than one prenatal test. After an unfavourable prenatal test outcome (with pregnancy termination) couples were engaged relatively quickly in a subsequent pregnancy and applied again for prenatal testing.

5. Discussion

During the last two decades major developments in DNA analysis have extended the technical possibilities of predictive and prenatal testing. Since testing with linked markers became available individuals at risk have been able to gain information about their genetic status with high probability before symptoms appear. In case of an uninformative predictive test result or for those who did not want to know their genetic status prenatal exclusion testing was offered to exclude carriership in offspring. Mutation detection provided more accurate DNA testing and brought new technologies such as PGD. However, the advances also introduced new complexities and dilemmas, e.g. the conflict of rights of 25% at-risk individuals versus 50% at-risk parents, and the controversial use of prenatal exclusion testing.

Despite the availability of full testing, prenatal exclusion testing is still requested by individuals at risk who do not want to know their own genetic status. Those individuals at risk choose to eventually terminate a pregnancy, while the fetus is only 50% at-risk of a late-onset disease, rather than knowing their own genetic status. It is clear from those cases and from case studies (see Chapter 2) that the choices in reproduction are personal and individual.

To date, systematic information about reproductive choices in persons at risk for HD is scarce. A few studies indicate the low uptake of prenatal diagnosis (Decruyenaere *et al.*, 1996; Maat-Kievit *et al.*, 1999; Simpson and Harper, 2001; Tolmie *et al.*, 1995), which appeared much lower than expected.

Table 10. Time interval between two consecutive prenatal tests, in relation with the test outcome of the previous prenatal test ($N = 41$ couples, centre level data)

Time interval	Unfavourable previous test result ($N = 46$)	Favourable previous test result ($N = 27$)
< 6 months	17	
6 months to 1 year	20	
1–2 years	5	9
2–3 years	3	7
> 3 years	1	11

The collaborative study presented here is one of the first to attempt to produce a large-scale investigation to increase knowledge and understanding about uptake and characteristics of prenatal testing for HD. In six European countries only 305 prenatal tests were reported between 1993 and 1998. In seven participating genetic centres 202 prenatal tests were reported between 1988 and 1999. These figures are designated as low in absolute terms, however, we did not assess their relative significance compared with the number of at-risk individuals in particular regions or countries. From the series in The Netherlands we know that 11% of the carriers tested (1987–1997) applied for prenatal testing (Maat-Kievit et al., 1999). These low figures were explained by the mean age (35 years) of the testees and the substantial number of testees with a completed family. Other explanations for the low uptake are difficulties in coping with pregnancy termination, ethical reservations about pregnancy termination for a late-onset disease, expected distress for future children having a parent at high risk and the hope for a cure for HD (Adam et al., 1993). The low uptake also stresses that the fear of a technological imperative is unfounded in prenatal testing. It is evident that most individuals clearly see the drawbacks of prenatal diagnosis and decide for other options.

When we compare the uptake rate of prenatal testing in the six countries the diversity is striking. Uptake in the UK and The Netherlands is high compared with the few prenatal tests in France and Greece. However, when we take into account the population of each country, the proportion of prenatal tests is highest in The Netherlands (90 prenatal tests/16 000 000 inhabitants = 5.63), followed by Belgium (2.92), the UK (2.62), Italy (0.33), Greece (0.18) and France (0.12). It is argued that historical or cultural differences or perhaps personality differences between northern and southern European populations may explain these differences in uptake, in particular concerning the views and beliefs about responsibility and autonomy in reproductive decision-making. Interestingly, one of the countries with the lowest uptake for prenatal testing for HD in our survey is Greece, a country with a record of near eradication of a common genetic disease (β-thalassaemia) as a result of widely accepted prenatal diagnosis (Chapter 5).

The relatively high number of at-risk individuals applying for prenatal testing and the high uptake rate for exclusion tests in the UK and Italy is another striking finding. These results may outline the influence of genetic counselling and counsellors and the diversity in communication of complex genetic information. It is possible that differences in the process of genetic counselling, e.g. in non-directiveness or in the amount or content of counselling, may have influenced the reproductive choices. It is also understandable that the technological advances in DNA testing may have affected the content and type of communicating reproductive options. In addition, professionals in genetic counselling may have welcomed the new options, whereas others may have reacted more reluctantly which may have influenced (unconsciously or unintentionally) their role or attitude in the process of genetic counselling. This issue does not imply right or wrong in genetic counselling, it just stresses the, perhaps underestimated and subtle differences in communication processes, which may contribute to the differences in uptake rate between genetic centres and countries.

As stated previously the use of prenatal exclusion testing is disputed. The results of this collaborative study show that there are a substantial number of at-risk individuals requesting prenatal exclusion tests. Therefore, their wish to exclude carriership in their offspring without clarifying their own risk should be acknowledged. It should also be noted that the long-term consequences of a pregnancy termination at 50% risk need careful consideration: in the long-term it may become obvious that the at-risk person is a non-carrier implicating that pregnancies have been terminated unnecessarily.

In addition to prenatal exclusion testing, full prenatal testing may be valued as a useful option by prospective parents who do not know their genetic status. Our study has shown that a minority of counsellees at risk deliberately chose this option. Some clinicians are hesitant about full prenatal testing in at-risk individuals because of the risk of finding dual or triple bad news. However, the chance of finding the gene in the fetus (implicating that the parent is a gene carrier as well) is only 25%, which may be more acceptable for some test applicants compared with the pros and cons of exclusion testing.

In brief, our study has shown that prenatal exclusion testing and full prenatal testing in at-risk individuals serve as valuable options and it is therefore suggested that full prenatal testing in at-risk individuals should be included in the international guidelines for predictive and prenatal testing (International Huntington Association and World Federation of Neurology Research Group on Huntington's Chorea, 1994). Guided exclusion testing was used rarely in this study, presumably because of the time-consuming aspects of this technique.

Another issue that arose from the results of this study is the entry of affected individuals into prenatal testing. The UK reported almost exclusively prenatal tests with affected prospective parents. Except for one case in Greece no affect-ed applicants were reported in the other four countries. This may have been caused by the absence of neurological evaluation of applicants before entering the prenatal test procedure. So, in those instances it is probably uncertain whether prenatal test applicants were affected or unaffected. In addition, it is argued that neurological examination is unnecessary or undesired, because the difference between an affected person and asymptomatic gene carrier is considered as relatively minor with respect to the future child.

Regarding the sex of the prospective parents we found a majority of females in The Netherlands; in the other countries the sexes were more equally distrib-uted. In the Dutch situation, it has been argued that females are more involved in reproductive choices than men. In addition, men may not want to burden their partners with prenatal testing or men and women may differ in coping strategies with respect to prenatal testing (Maat-Kievit et al., 1999).

The results regarding repeated prenatal testing are very interesting. It was found that about one-third of the couples applied between two and five times for prenatal testing. This finding suggests that prenatal diagnosis is carefully chosen by a relatively small group of individuals at risk. Perhaps the applicants with repeated prenatal tests are a self-selected group who feel well prepared for prenatal testing and eventual pregnancy termination (see also Codori *et al.*, 1994). From a Dutch pilot study we know that prenatal test applicants had already discussed the option of prenatal testing a long time before a pregnancy was established and even before the parent was tested positively (Zoeteweij *et al.*, 1997), indicating long-term preparation which may facilitate adaptation after prenatal test disclosure (Dudok de Wit *et al.*, 1998). This may emphasize that information about prenatal options should be provided at an early stage, e.g. during the counselling sessions of predictive testing procedures.

The high representation of repeated prenatal tests also implies that many applicants adhere to their initial choice and find it difficult to make changes in reproductive options. It should be noted that choosing another reproductive option might introduce different risk statuses for children in one family with possible adverse psychological consequences. Adam *et al.* (1993) stated that it is advisable for couples to consider all the options in each pregnancy and make an attempt to choose independent of earlier strategies.

The time lapse after an unfavourable prenatal test result appeared to be short, expressing the high time pressure on high-risk applicants or mutation carriers who approach the age of onset of the disease. In addition, this group may have been well prepared for pregnancy termination and therefore need little time to recover. They also may attempt to escape from distress or deny their loss with the creation of a new pregnancy.

Finally, some limitations of the study should be noted. First, there is the limitation of retrospective data collection including primarily quantitative data. The case presentations presented by Jacopini *et al.* (Chapter 2) have significantly enriched the data. Nevertheless, it is obvious that prospective data would have strengthened the study design. Second, there was a substantial amount of missing data for some variables (in particular the age and sex of prospective parents) in some centres, which may weaken some of the results. Third, we have to take into account that the content and amount of prenatal test procedures may differ from one country to another and even from one centre to another in the same country. Discussions between the co-authors of this European collaborative study have indeed revealed that counselling procedures in the six countries are similar in some respects (e.g. consensus on risk information, information about HD), but also differ (e.g. different professionals involved in the counselling procedure, different procedures for test disclosure) with possible large implications for the uptake for prenatal diagnosis.

Despite these limitations, this study has shown that different options in prenatal testing are requested and should be acknowledged as valuable options for small subsets of individuals. The increase in technical possibilities implicates an increase in the responsibilities and skills of professionals in genetic counselling to communicate carefully and sensitively about these possibilities. Counsellors and counsellees should also bear in mind that the facts of today may be outdated tomorrow because of new technological advances.

With the application of expert knowledge in communication skills and decision counselling the focus of *genetic* counselling will shift more and more to genetic *counselling* which will guarantee the optimal service for individuals applying for prenatal testing.

Acknowledgements

The authors explicitly acknowledge the contribution of the many persons in the participating genetic centres, without whom this study would not have been possible. In Belgium: Dr M. Decruyenaere, Mrs T. Cloostermans, Mrs A. Boogaerts, Professor J.P. Fryns (Center for Human Genetics, Leuven), Professor J. Dumon (Dienst voor erfelijkheidsonderzoek en advies, Antwerpen), Professor Y. Gillerot (Département de Génétique Médicale, Loverval), Professor A. de Paepe, Mrs I. Delvaux (Dienst Medische Genetica, Gent), Professor I. Liebaers (Dienst Medische Genetica, Bruxelles), Professor M. Abramovicz (Centre de Génétique, Bruxelles), Professor A. Verloes (Service de Génétique Humaine, Liège), Professor C. Verellen (Centre de Génétique Médicale, Bruxelles). In the UK: Mrs R. Glew, Dr R. Harper (Institute of Medical Genetics, Cardiff), the members of the UK Huntington's Disease Prediction Consortium. In The Netherlands: Dr J.A. Maat-Kievit, Professor M.H. Breuning, Dr M. Losekoot, Professor B. Bakker (Dept of Human and Clinical Genetics, Leiden), Mrs M.N. Ané, Professor R.A.C. Roos (Dept of Neurology, Leiden), Dutch Working Group on Huntington's Disease, in collaboration with: Afdeling Erfelijkheidsadvisering Academisch Medisch Centrum Amsterdam (Professor N.J. Leschot), Afdeling Klinische Genetica Vrije Universiteit Amsterdam (Professor L.P. ten Kate), Afdeling Erfelijkheidsvoor lichting Rijksuniversiteit Groningen (Dr J.A. van Essen), Afdeling Erfelijkheids voorlichting Stichting Klinische Genetica ZO Nederland Maastricht (Dr C. Schrandel-Stumpel), Afdeling Klinische Genetica Radboud Ziekenhuis Nijmegen (Professor H. Brunner), Divisie Medische Genetica Universitair Medisch Centrum Utrecht (Professor D. Lindhout), Afdeling Klinische Genetica Leids Universitair Medisch Centrum Leiden (Professor M.H. Breuning). In France: Professor J. Feingold, Mrs M. Garguilo, Mrs T. Carpecchi, Dr K. Lahlou (Hôpital de la Salpêtrière, Paris). In Italy: Dr M. Frontali (Istituto di Medicina Sperimentale CNR, Roma), Professor B. Brambati (Istituto Ostetrico-Ginecologico 'L. Mangiagalli', Milano), Dr P. Mandich (Dipartemento Oncologia, Biologia e Genetica, Genova), Professor A. Renieri (Istituto di Genetica Medica Università di Siena), Dr M. Genuardi (Istituto di Genetica Medica Università Cattolica Sacro Cuore, Roma), Professor G. Novelli (Cattedra di Genetica Medica Università Tor Vergata, Roma), Dr M. Ferrari (Biologia Moleculae Clinica Ospedale San Raffaele, Milano), Professor E. Calzolari (Genetica Umana Università di Ferrara, Ferrara). In Greece: Professor C. Papageorgiou, Professor M. Dalakas, Professor D. Vassilopoulos, Dr C. Voumvourakis, Dr M. Pana, Mrs S. Pomoni (Dept of Neurology, University of Athens), Professor D. Loukopoulos, Mrs K. Palioniko (1st Dept of Internal Medicine, University of Athens), Professor C. Metaxotou, Dr S. Youroukos (1st Dept of Pediatrics, University of Athens), Assoc. Professor A. Antsaklis (1st Dept of Gynecology and Obstetrics, University of Athens), Professor A. Plaitakis, Dr M. Tzagournissakis (Dept of Neurology, University of Crete, Herakleion).

References

Adam, S., Wiggins, S., Whyte, P., et al (1993) Five year study of prenatal testing for Huntington disease: demand, attitudes and psychological assessment. *J. Med. Genet.* **30:** 549–556.

Almqvist, E., Adam, S., Bloch, M., et al (1997) Risk reversals in predictive testing for Huntington disease. *Am. J. Hum. Genet.* **61:** 945–952.

Almqvist, E., Bloch M., Brinkman, R., Craufurd, D. and Hayden, M.R. (1999) A worldwide assessment of suicide, suicide attempts or psychiatric hospitalization after predictive testing for Huntington disease. *Am. J. Hum. Genet.* **64:** 1293–1304.

Bloch, M., Adam, S., Wiggins, S., Huggins, M. and Hayden, M.R. (1992) Predictive testing for Huntington disease in Canada. The experience of those receiving an increased risk. *Am. J. Med. Genet.* **42:** 499.

Codori, A.M. and Brandt, J. (1994) Psychological costs and benefits of predictive testing for Huntington's disease. *Am. J. Med. Genet.* **54:** 174–184.

Codori, A.M., Hanson, R. and Brandt, J. (1994) Self-selection in predictive testing for Huntington's disease. *Am. J. Med. Genet.* **54:** 167–173.

Decruyenaere, M, Evers-Kiebooms, G., Boogaerts, A., Cassiman, J.J., Cloostermans, T., Demyttenaere, K., Dom, R., Fryns, J.-P. and Van den Berghe H. (1996) Prediction of psychological functioning one year after the predictive test for Huntington's disease and the impact of the test result on reproductive decision making. *J. Med. Genet.* **33:** 737–743.

Dudok de Wit, A.C., Tibben, A., Duivenvoorden, H.J., Niermeyer, M.F., Passchier, J. and the other members of the Rotterdam/Leiden Genetics Workgroup (1998) Predicting adaptation to presymptomatic DNA testing for late onset disorders: who will experience distress? *J. Med. Genet.* **35:** 745–754.

Evers-Kiebooms, G., Nys, K., Harper, P., Zoeteweij, M., Dürr, A., Jacopini, G., Yapijakis, C. and Simpson, S. Predictive DNA-testing for Huntington's disease and reproductive decision making: a European collaborative study (submitted).

Evers-Kiebooms, G., Welkenhuysen, M., Claes, E., Decruyenaere, M. and Denayer L. (2000) The psychological complexity of predictive testing for late onset neurogenetic diseases and hereditary cancers. *Soc. Sci. Med.* **51:** 831–841.

Frets, P.G., Duivenvoorden, H.J., Verhage, F., Niermeyer, M.F., V d Berge, S.M.M. and Galjaard, H. (1990) Factors influencing the reproductive decisions after genetic counselling. *Am. J. Med. Genet.* **35:** 496–502.

Gusella, J.F., Wexler, N.S., Conneally, P.M., et al (1983) A polymorphic DNA marker genetically linked to Huntington's disease. *Nature* **306:** 234–238.

Harper, P. (1996) *Huntington's Disease.* Saunders, London.

Horowitz, M., Sundin, E., Zanko, A. and Lauer, R. (2001) Coping with grim news from genetic tests. *Psychosomatics* **42:** 100–105.

Huggins, M., Bloch, M., Wiggins, S., et al (1992) Predictive testing for Huntington's disease in Canada: adverse effects and unexpected results in those receiving a decreased risk. *Am. J. Med. Genet.* **42:** 508–515.

Huntington, G. (1872) On chorea. *Medl Surg. Reporter* **26:** 320–321.

Huntington Disease Collaborative Research Group (1993) A novel gene containing a trinucleotide repeat that is expanded in Huntington's disease chromosomes. *Cell* **72:** 971–983.

International Huntington Association and World Federation of Neurology Research Group on Huntington's Chorea (1994) Guidelines for the molecular genetics predictive test in Huntington's disease. *J. Med. Genet.* **31:** 555–559.

Kelly, T.E., Allinson, P., McGlennan, R.C., Baker, J. and Bao, Y. (1999) Expansion of a 27 CAG repeat allele into a symptomatic Huntington disease-producing allele. *Am. J. Med. Genet.* **87:** 91–92.

Lawson, K., Wiggins, S., Green, T., Adam, S., Bloch, M. and Hayden, M.R. (1996) Adverse psychological events occurring in the first year after predictive testing for Huntington's disease. The Canadian Collaborative Study Predictive Testing. *J. Med. Genet.* **33:** 856–862.

Maat-Kievit, A., Vegter-van der Vlis, M., Zoeteweij, M., Losekoot, M., van Haeringen, A., Kanhai, H. and Roos, R. (1999) Experience in prenatal testing for Huntington's disease in The Netherlands: procedures, results and guidelines (1987–1997). *Prenat. Diagn.* **99:** 450–457.

Mastromauro, C., Myers, R.H. and Berkman, B. (1987) Attitudes toward presymptomatic testing in Huntington's disease. *Am. J. Med. Genet.* **26:** 271–282.

Simpson, S.A. and Harding A.E. (1993) Predictive testing for Huntington's disease: after the gene. The United Kingdom Huntington's Disease Prediction Consortium. *J. Med. Genet.* **30:** 1036–1038.

Simpson, S.A. and Harper, P.S. (2001) Prenatal testing for Huntington's disease: experience within the UK 1994–1998. *J. Med. Genet.* **38:** 333–335.

Tibben, A., Duivenvoorden, H.J., Niermeyer, M.F., Vegter-van der Vlis, M., Roos, R.A.C. and Verhage, F. (1994) Psychological effects of presymptomatic DNA testing for Huntington's disease in the Dutch program. *Psychosom. Med.* **56:** 526–532.

Tibben, A., Timman, R., Bannink, E.C. and Duivenvoorden, H.J. (1997) Three-year follow-up after presymptomatic testing for Huntington disease in tested individuals and partners. *Health Psychol.* **16:** 20–35.75

Tolmie, J.L., Davidson, H.R., May, H.M., McIntosh, K., Paterson, J.S. and Smith, B. (1995) The prenatal exclusion test for Huntington's disease: experience in the West of Scotland, 1986–1993. *J. Med. Genet.* **32:** 97–101.

Tyler, A., Quarrell, O., Lazarou, L.P., Meredith, A.L. and Harper, P.S. (1990) Exclusion testing in pregnancy for Huntington's disease. *J. Med. Genet.* **27:** 488–495.

Williams, J.K., Schutte, D.L., Evers, C. and Holkup, P.A. (2000) Redefinition: coping with normal results from predictive gene testing for neurodegenerative disorders. *Res. Nurs. Health* **23:** 260–269.

Zoeteweij, M.W., Geerinck-Vercammen, C.R., Maat-Kievit, J.A., Losekoot, M., Kanhai, H.H.H. and van Haeringen, A. (1997) Prenatal testing for Huntington's disease: first results of a psychological follow-up study in the Netherlands. *Genet. Counsell.* **8:** 147–148.

4

Reproductive history after predictive testing for Huntington's disease: a European collaborative study

Gerry Evers-Kiebooms, Kurt Nys, Peter S. Harper,
Moniek W. Zoeteweij, Alexandra Dürr, Gioia Jacopini,
Christos Yapijakis and Sheila A. Simpson

1. Introduction

Huntington's disease (HD) was the first late-onset disease for which predictive testing became available and, moreover, it has often been used as a paradigm for other autosomal dominant late-onset neurogenetic diseases. This chapter focuses on reproductive decision-making after predictive testing for HD.

Huntington's disease is a currently untreatable progressive neuropsychiatric disorder, characterized by involuntary movements, neuropsychological defects and personality changes. The mean age at onset is about 40 years. Symptoms progress slowly with death occurring an average of 15 years after disease onset. Huntington's disease is inherited as an autosomal dominant trait, with the gene localized on the short arm of chromosome 4. In March 1993, the Huntington gene was isolated containing an expanded and unstable trinucleotide repeat (CAG) in HD patients (Huntington's Disease Collaborative Research Group, 1993). The localization and subsequent identification of the gene resulted in the offer of a predictive DNA test to asymptomatic persons belonging to families with HD. In a recent article, Harper *et al.* (2000), on behalf of the UK Huntington's Disease Prediction Consortium, stated 'the normal range was classified as up to 30 repeats, with 39 or more repeats as abnormal, the small intervening number being considered as "equivocal"' (p. 568). Persons

Prenatal Testing for Late-Onset Neurogenetic Diseases, edited by G. Evers-Kiebooms,
M. W. Zoeteweij and P. S. Harper

with a predictive test result in the latter category are also called persons with an intermediate allele; this result is quite exceptional (1.5% of the persons with a predictive test in the UK in the period 1988–1997).

About 15 years ago the introduction of a predictive DNA test for HD was an important milestone in medical history, as well as a challenge for families and professionals. In the meantime, increasing knowledge about the human genome has resulted in the availability of predictive and prenatal tests for several other neurogenetic diseases (Chapters 5, 11 and 13). The specific nature of predictive tests for late-onset neurogenetic diseases and the need for careful protocols and a multidisciplinary approach has already been discussed in Evers-Kiebooms (Chapter 1). Because of the particular nature of predictive tests for (currently) untreatable late-onset diseases, a large amount of international debate and consultation preceded the implementation of the first predictive DNA tests in clinical practice. Successive guidelines elaborated by the International Huntington Association and the World Federation of Neurology (1994) is an example in this context. In the meantime, the multidisciplinary approach for predictive testing for HD has been a model for other neurogenetic diseases.

We start with a brief review of the uptake for predictive testing, paying particular attention to 'family planning' as a reason to apply for predictive testing, as well as to intentions to use prenatal testing. For a review on the impact of predictive testing on the psychological well-being of testees and their family we refer to Evers-Kiebooms et al. (2000). The major part of this chapter presents the results of a systematic European collaborative study, involving seven genetic centres in six countries (Belgium, France, Italy, Greece, The Netherlands and the UK) regarding the impact of the predictive test result upon subsequent reproduction and the uptake for prenatal testing in the group of carriers of the Huntington mutation. Systematic studies on this topic are lacking, notwithstanding the fact that predictive testing for HD and prenatal testing for HD as two separate issues have received a lot of attention. For the results of a systematic European collaborative study on prenatal testing we refer to Chapter 3. For overall data on predictive and prenatal testing for HD in other European countries and in North America we refer respectively to Chapters 5 and 13.

2. The role of family planning as a reason for predictive testing and the intentions to use prenatal testing

All over the world the proportion of persons applying for predictive testing is smaller than might be expected based on intentions and attitudes before the availability of the test: the uptake rate is estimated between 5 and 20% (cf. Chapter 1).

Decruyenaere et al. (1997) assessed the perceived benefits or reasons for taking the test and the perceived barriers to taking the test in tested and untested persons belonging to the same sibships. The most important benefits or reasons for taking the test are: the need for certainty or relief from uncertainty, making reproductive decisions, informing their children about their risk for HD and making decisions on practical matters (financial, employment). Important barriers to the test are: the anticipated inability to cope with an unfavourable test result (fear for a bad test result), the feeling that important decisions do not have to depend on a test result, being happier when not knowing than with the certainty of a bad result, the lack of a treatment, concern about the reaction of their children and partner. These reported benefits and barriers are compatible with the findings in other studies (Quaid and Morris, 1993; Van der Steenstraten *et al.*, 1994). In some countries, concern about life insurance is an additional barrier to taking the test (Harper, 1996). Of course the motivation to have or not have a predictive test is very complex (often there is more than one reason or motive) and consists of conscious and unconscious motives. It is important to keep in mind that in most surveys or other studies only the conscious motives expressed or indicated by the persons at risk for HD are taken into account. In most centres around the world which reported their data, the two major motives for requesting predictive testing are 'certainty for their own future' and 'family planning'. With respect to the latter, the findings in many centres around the world (Adam *et al.*, 1993; Decruyenaere *et al.*, 1997; Evers-Kiebooms *et al.*, 1996; Schulman *et al.*, 1996; Tolmie *et al.*, 1995; Tyler *et al.*, 1990) illustrate that carriers of the Huntington mutation with a desire for children are confronted with new decision difficulties and an additional emotional burden. They have the following options: refraining from having children, taking the risk of having a child with the Huntington mutation, using prenatal diagnosis, adoption, artificial insemination with donor sperm, *in vitro* fertilization (IVF) with donor eggs and more recently in a small number of centres in the world preimplantation genetic diagnosis (PGD). The use of PGD for late-onset neurogenetic diseases is discussed by Geraedts and Liebaers (Chapter 7). The psychological cost of this option is discussed in Evers-Kiebooms *et al.* (1996) and is also illustrated in the case presentations by de Die and Heurckmans (Chapter 8).

There have been very few systematic studies on reproductive choices in HD families following the introduction of predictive and prenatal DNA testing. Moreover, there are almost no studies on reproductive choices following a predictive test result. In Manchester (Craufurd *et al.*, 1989), 81% of the 109 'potential users' said they would request prenatal diagnosis if pregnant, whereas only 3 couples had a prenatal test. In Wales (Tyler *et al.*, 1990), 17% of 90 couples referred to the genetic centre for information about exclusion testing in the period 1986–1989, had one or more prenatal exclusion tests. After a positive test result all pregnancies were terminated. The most important reason for prenatal diagnosis not being accepted by the other couples was objection to pregnancy termination for HD. Adam *et al.* (1993) reported on 'intentions to use' prenatal diagnosis and 'use' of prenatal testing in the group of subjects who had entered the Canadian Collaborative Study on predictive testing before September 1991. Overall 43% had the intention to use prenatal testing if they or their spouse were pregnant. During the study period, 18% of the 38 couples who did not receive a decreased risk and who had one or more pregnancies in the study period used prenatal diagnosis. All but one increased risk pregnancies were terminated. The most frequent reason given for declining prenatal testing was the hope that a cure would be found in time (about 80% of the candidates). Other reasons were: reluctance to terminate the pregnancy, concern about the safety of the prenatal procedure and wanting to determine own status before deciding about prenatal testing. Subjects who already had children and practising members of a religious organization were less likely to choose prenatal diagnosis. Some couples in the study of Adam *et al.* (1993) felt that there was a 'technological imperative' to use the prenatal test in every pregnancy. After a first prenatal diagnosis, couples could only justify the initial use of prenatal testing if they continued to use the same technology in further pregnancies. In this way, several couples had repeated prenatal diagnoses with a lot of psychological suffering after successive losses. However, these feelings of suffering may be denied and couples may experience it differently, e.g. as an obligation or a responsibility they have to take. In-depth counselling should free individuals from any 'technological imperative' and allow them to make independent choices in every pregnancy (cf. also the case presentations in Chapter 2). Tolmie *et al.* (1995) reported that in the period 1986–1993, 10 couples underwent one or more exclusion tests in west Scotland. When the risk was increased, one-third of the pregnancies were continued: the mother had made a 'last minute' decision not to undergo the planned termination. In 26 of the 43 couples applying for prenatal tests in The Netherlands before 1998 prior predictive testing showed that one of the partners was a carrier of the Huntington mutation. These 26 couples are 11% of the total group of tested carriers, whatever their age at the time of predictive testing (Maat-Kievit *et al.*, 1999). The study of Decruyenaere *et al.* (1996) revealed that, one year after the predictive test, about one-third of the carriers with reproductive plans refrained from having children, one-third chose to have prenatal diagnosis and one-third was undecided about future pregnancies. Another striking finding in the same study: a few women had stopped contraception in the pretest period, some weeks before receiving a predictive test result. One of them was pregnant before she got her result. The risky contraceptive behaviour of these women may be an expression of their ambivalence towards reproduction in this situation. On the one hand, they had a strong desire for children, but on the other hand, they felt reluctant to have children with prenatal diagnosis, or without prenatal diagnosis. The 'unconscious' contraceptive risk-taking may be an attempt to escape from the responsibility to take a personal decision (Lippman-Hand and Fraser, 1979). This shows that reproductive decisions in a situation of increased genetic risk are very complex and subject to emotional and unconscious processes.

A very difficult situation arises when parents decide to continue with the pregnancy when the fetus is carrier of the Huntington mutation. Indeed, the child to be born may later in life be harmed by this information. It cannot be excluded that the known carrier status may have a negative impact on the child's upbringing: either by spoiling or overprotecting or by neglecting the child. Moreover, the child's right not to know is already violated before his birth. All these issues should receive attention during counselling before the parents engage in a pregnancy with prenatal diagnosis.

Results of a survey assessing the uptake of prenatal testing for HD world-wide, carried out in close collaboration with the World Federation of the Neurology Research Group on Huntington's Disease, revealed that the uptake of prenatal testing is low, but that the results largely vary between different countries and between different centres within a country (Evers-Kiebooms, 1997). The prediction of Hayden *et al.* (1995) that the demand for prenatal testing would further decrease in the future because of the optimism about a potential treatment has become true in some countries. Recently, Hayden (2001) reported that not a single prenatal test for HD was performed in British Columbia during the previous 5 years.

3. A European collaborative study assessing the reproductive history after predictive testing for HD

3.1 Introduction

As already mentioned, systematic studies about the factors influencing the decision to utilize prenatal testing for HD are rather scarce. Studies on small samples, studies with short-term follow-up and case studies have mainly been reported in scientific journals. To obtain more insight into the psychosocial, ethical and legal complexity of prenatal testing for HD a European collabora-tive, multidisciplinary study was set up with seven participants from genetic centres, a partner with expertise in the legal aspects of genetic testing, a part-ner with expertise in the ethical aspects of genetic testing and a partner from the European Huntington Association. This study was carried out in the con-text of a European Commission (EC)-funded project (BIOMED-project N° ERB BMH4-CT98–3926). The objectives of the European project are given in Chapter 1. The European project also created a forum for the discussion of all aspects of prenatal testing for late-onset neurogenetic disease during a multi-disciplinary BIOMED meeting, which was organized at the end of 2000 in Leuven, with a very active involvement of delegates from Huntington Associations from the majority of EC countries.

It is the main aim of this chapter to describe and analyse the reproductive history of carriers of the Huntington mutation compared with non-carriers. Prenatal diagnosis and, more recently, PGD can be considered as import-ant options among others in the context of reproductive decision-making of car-riers of the Huntington mutation. Evers-Kiebooms *et al.* (1996) clearly expressed the need for an adequate counselling context, to ensure free informed reproductive decision-making for persons belonging to families con-fronted with HD.

3.2 Methodology

Seven genetic centres from six European countries took an active part in the collection of the data in this European collaborative study: Leuven, Leiden, Cardiff, Aberdeen, Paris, Rome and Athens. Six centres were project partners right from the start. The genetic centre at Aberdeen was involved after the first year of the project on behalf of the UK Huntington Disease Prediction Consortium. Two types of data were collected by the seven genetic centres: data about individual prenatal tests for HD at centre level and at country level (type 1 data) and data about the reproductive history of persons who had a predictive test for HD (type 2 data). The type 1 data (all prenatal tests performed) at centre- and at country level are discussed in Chapter 3. A selection of data from the first part of the European collaborative study is discussed by Simpson *et al.* (submitted).

Here we focus exclusively on the reproductive history of persons who had a predictive test for HD (type 2 data) in each of the seven participating centres. It is important to keep in mind that most of these centres have used careful predictive test protocols and a multidisciplinary approach (Chapter 1) since the start of their predictive test programme. The study group in each of the seven centres consisted of persons who had a predictive test and who met the following criteria: (i) the testee had to be 45 or younger at the time of the communication of the test result, (ii) the testee had to be tested and counselled in one of the seven centres (no extension to the country level), and (iii) the communication of the predictive test result had to be done after 1992 and before 1999.

For the systematic and accurate collection of the type 2 data on reproductive decision-making after predictive testing a three-page questionnaire was developed. Information on the following topics was sought: (i) date and result of the predictive test, (ii) sociodemographic data, (iii) reasons for predictive testing based on the files from the pretest period, (iv) information about the last contact with the testee, (v) pregnancies, (vi) adoptions, (vii) presence of a pregnancy at the time of communicating the test result, (viii) perception of completeness of the family, and (ix) intentions for PGD. For most topics multiple-choice questions were used. Information was usually retrieved from the files, which in principle contained data from the post-test follow-up sessions, by professionals from the genetic centres. When feasible, the testee was contacted by the genetic centre to update the data, hereby always paying attention to the 'well-being' of the testee and respecting testees' choice to have no further follow-up contact (the latter was only the case for a small minority). In the genetic centre at Leiden a slightly different approach was used and only the subgroup of testees participating in another ongoing study and meeting the eligibility criteria for this study were involved in this part of the European collaborative study.

All the completed forms were mailed to Leuven, where the data were centralized and analysed using the SAS package for the statistical analysis of data. Respect for the privacy of the testees was ensured by anonymizing all the data before sending them to the coordinating centre. There was only an identification number on the forms sent to Leuven. A critical discussion of preliminary analyses and intermediate evaluations of the progress of the different aspects of the project took place during workshops with all project participants. A selection of data from the second part of the European collaborative study is discussed by Evers-Kiebooms *et al.* (2002).

3.3 Results

A description of the study group

Age, carrier status and motives for applying for predictive testing.   The total study group consisted of 453 testees: 180 carriers, 271 non-carriers and 2 testees with an intermediate allele. The reproductive history for the two individuals with an intermediate allele is discussed separately. *Table 1* gives an overview of the results of the predictive tests per centre. All the participating centres had more predictive tests with a 'no carrier' result than with a 'carrier' result. In the total group, 60% of the testees were non-carriers and 40% were asymptomatic carriers of the Huntington mutation. The ratio favourable/unfavourable predictive test results was similar in the participating centres.

Table 1. Composition of the study group: centre and carrier status*

Centre	Carrier	Non-carrier
Leuven	28	39
Leiden	19	39
Cardiff	23	37
Aberdeen	29	32
Paris	38	46
Rome	10	19
Athens	33	59
Total group	180	271

*Two testees had an intermediate allele and were not included.

The distribution of the year of the communication of the predictive test result is compatible with the general trend of increased uptake in the first year after the identification of the gene (*Fig. 1*). The lower numbers for the later years are

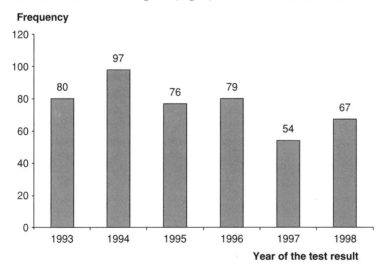

Figure 1. Year of communication of the predictive test result ($N = 453$).

due in part to the fact that predictive testing steadily became available in an increasing number of genetic centres in five of the six participating countries. There were slightly more female (58%) than male (42%) testees. The mean age of the testees ($N = 453$) was 31.5 years (SD, 7.03; range, 18–45). The information per centre is given in *Table 2*. The majority of testees (77%) were in a stable relationship at the time of the communication of the test result. The mean age of the partner of the testee ($N = 298$) was 33.3 years (SD, 7.67; range, 18–61). Overall, about half of the testees were aged 31 years or younger when they received the predictive test result.

The most frequently mentioned reason for applying for predictive testing (expressed in the pretest period) was 'having certainty' or 'getting rid of uncertainty': 81% of testees expressed this reason as a major motive to apply for predictive testing for HD. 'Reproductive decision-making' was mentioned by 38% of testees as a major reason and 'informing the children' by 28%. Eleven per cent mentioned other motives for predictive testing. The percentages do not add up to 100% because there was an opportunity to indicate more than one major reason. Taking into account the mean age of the testees at the time of the communication of the predictive test result, the percentage of testees mentioning family planning as a motive appears rather low. As might be expected, there is a significant negative correlation between the age of the testee and the expression of reproductive decision-making as a motive for having a predictive test ($r = -0.31$; $p < 0.001$): the older the testee the less frequent reproductive decision-making was mentioned as one of the main motives to apply for predictive testing. A similar negative correlation was found with the age of the partner of the testee ($r = -0.38$; $p < 0.001$). Almost 70% of the testees with reproductive decision-making as a motive for applying for predictive testing were aged between 20 and 30 years and about 30% between 30 and 40 years (only 3 testees with reproductive decision-making as motive to apply for predictive testing were not between 20 and 40 years old).

Pregnancies before communication of the predictive test result. Details of the number of pregnancies before communication of the predictive test

Table 2. Mean age of the testee at the time of the communication of the predictive test result per centre ($N = 453$)

Centre	Mean	SD (range)
Leuven	29.6	6.9 (18–45)
Leiden	32.3	7.3 (18–45)
Cardiff	33.0	7.4 (19–45)
Aberdeen	31.0	7.7 (18–45)
Paris	32.2	6.7 (18–45)
Rome	31.3	6.1 (19–41)
Athens	29.9	6.7 (20–45)
Total group	31.5	7.0 (18–45)

Table 3. Number of pregnancies per testee *before* the communication of the predictive test result*

Number of pregnancies	Carrier group (%) (N = 180)	Non-carrier group (%) (N = 271)	Total group (%) (N = 451)
0	47	51	50
1	21	16	18
2	22	20	20
3	6	9	8
4	4	4	4
	100	100	100

*The two testees with an intermediate allele are not included here or in the subsequent analyses.

result can be found in *Table 3*. This information is given for the group who were revealed to be carriers and the group who were revealed to be non-carriers, as well as for the total group independent of the predictive test result. About half of the carriers and half of the non-carriers already had one or more pregnancies before applying for predictive testing. Overall, there were 442 pregnancies before the predictive test. One hundred and eighty carriers of the Huntington gene had 177 pregnancies, 271 non-carriers had 265 pregnancies. These pregnancies resulted in the birth of 388 children, 32 miscarriages and 22 terminations without prenatal testing (in this type of survey no more information is available about these terminations). In the total study group nine testees had one or more pregnancies with prenatal diagnosis for HD before the communication of the predictive test result (13 prenatal exclusion tests).

The number of pregnancies before the communication of the result of the predictive test was significantly correlated with the presence of reproductive decision-making as a reason to apply for predictive testing ($r = -0.31$; $p < 0.001$): as might be expected the more pregnancies there were before the predictive test, the less frequent reproductive decision-making was mentioned as a motive for applying for predictive testing. In the group without any pregnancy before the predictive test the number of testees mentioning reproductive decision-making as a reason to apply for predictive testing was comparable with the number of testees not mentioning reproductive decision-making in the pretest period.

The length of the follow-up interval after the communication of the predictive test result.   For more than two-thirds of the study group the most recent contact with the testee took place in 1999 (47%) or 2000 (21%) (*Fig. 2*). The follow-up period was calculated as the difference between the date of the communication of the predictive test result and the reported date of the last contact in the returned questionnaire. For almost half of the testees (48%) the follow-up period was 3 years or longer (*Table 4*). Owing to the design of the study the maximum follow-up interval was 7 years. For 19% of the testees the follow-up

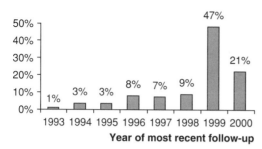

Figure 2. Percentage distribution of the year of the most recent contact with the testee ($N = 448$).

interval was less than 1 year, for 19% the follow-up interval was between 1 and 2 years and 13% had a follow-up interval between 2 and 3 years. Although a follow-up interval of 3 years or longer for about half of the group is not optimal it seems a satisfactory start for studying the reproductive history of the testees. However, it is important to realize that the families should not yet be considered as 'complete'.

For 89% of the testees the last follow-up contact was initiated by the genetic centre for the purpose of this study or for another reason and in 11% by the testee (frequency missing = 19). Sixty-nine per cent of the testees were contacted by a member of the team involved in pretest and/or post-test counselling (frequency missing = 51). This person belonging to the team was mostly a geneticist (33%), a social worker or social nurse (19%), or a psychologist (14%). In 70 questionnaires (13%) information about the profession of the person who contacted the testee was missing.

Reproductive history after the communication of the predicitve test result
An overall picture of post predictive test reproduction. The number of pregnancies after the communication of the predictive test result is shown in *Table 5*: 103 of the 451 testees reported one or more pregnancies. These 142 pregnancies resulted in the birth of 104 children, 22 miscarriages and 16 terminations. In the group of carriers 26/180 (14%) had one or more pregnancies. As might be expected the percentage of non-carriers with one or more pregnancies is much higher: 77/271 (28%) had one or more pregnancies. For the 40 pregnancies in the carrier group 24 prenatal tests for HD were performed: 9 prenatal tests had a favourable result and 15 an unfavourable. It can be derived

Table 4. Length of the follow-up period after the communication of the predictive test result

Follow-up period	Testees (%) ($N = 453$)
Less than 1 year	19
Between 1 and 2 years	19
Between 2 and 3 years	13
More than 3 years	48
	100

Table 5. An overall picture of post predictive test reproduction as a function of carrier status
($N = 451$)*

Number of pregnancies	Carrier (%) ($N = 180$)	Non-carrier (%) ($N = 271$)
0	85	72
1	9	22
2	4	3
3	1	3
6	1	0
	100	100

*Ongoing pregnancies at the time of the communication of the
test result were considered as pregnancies occurring in the pretest
period.

from Table 6 that 15 of the 26 carriers with one or more pregnancies had one
or more prenatal tests. Twelve pregnancies in the carrier group resulted in the
birth of a child, without a prenatal test. There were three miscarriages in this
group and one preimplantation genetic diagnosis.

*Reproductive history of carriers and non-carriers as a function of the presence
or absence of family planning as a motive in the pretest period.* By comparing the post predictive test reproductive history of carriers and non-carriers it is
obvious that the former group is less inclined to engage in a pregnancy.
However, it is very important to look at the data in a more 'refined' way, hereby
taking into account 'reproductive decision-making' as a motive for predictive
testing. Therefore we split the total group into four subgroups based on two
variables: (i) predictive test result, and (ii) mentioning reproductive decision-
making as a major motive in the pretest period. The results are shown in
Table 6. In the group of carriers who mentioned reproductive decision-making as a motive for predictive testing for HD in the pretest period ($N = 57$)
18 persons (32%) had pregnancies after the predictive test. The total number of pregnancies of these 18 persons was 31. Ten persons had one pregnancy, six had two, one had three, and one person had six post predictive test
pregnancies. Eleven carriers had one or more pregnancies with prenatal
diagnosis. Seven testees had none of their pregnancies tested (five testees
with one and two with two pregnancies). For the total of 31 pregnancies in
the carrier group 20 prenatal tests were performed. The 20 prenatal tests
that were performed in the carrier group resulted in 8 favourable results and
12 unfavourable results. All pregnancies with an unfavourable prenatal test
result were terminated. In seven pregnancies no prenatal test was performed.
Three pregnancies resulted in a miscarriage and one pregnancy occurred
after IVF and PGD.

When we focus on the subgroup of carriers with at least one prenatal diagnosis after predictive testing the following patterns are present. Ten carriers or
their spouse had a prenatal test in every pregnancy after the communication of
the predictive test result. In this group of ten testees, five testees had one

Table 6. Reproduction of carriers and non-carriers of the Huntington mutation as a function of the presence or absence of reproductive decision making as a motive for applying for predictive testing in the pretest period

	Carriers (N = 180)	Non-carriers (N = 271)	Total (N = 451)
Reproductive motive (N = 171)			
No. testees	57	114	171
No. testees with pregnancies	18	64	82
No. pregnancies	31	88	119
No. births (with PGD)	16 (1)	68	84
No. miscarriages	3	19	22
No. terminations	12	1	13
No. testees with prenatal tests	11		
No. prenatal tests	20		20
No. favourable result	8		8
No. unfavourable result	12		12
No reproductive motive (N = 280)			
No. testees	123	157	280
No. testees with pregnancies	8	13	21
No. pregnancies	9	14	23
No. births	6	14	20
No. miscarriages	0	0	0
No. terminations	3	0	3
No. testees with prenatal tests	4		4
No. prenatal tests	4		4
No. favourable result	1		1
No. unfavourable result	3		3

pregnancy, four had two and one had three pregnancies tested with prenatal testing. One testee had a more complicated pattern of performed prenatal tests. This testee had six pregnancies after the communication of the predictive test result. After an unfavourable prenatal test result in the first pregnancy, a miscarriage in the second pregnancy, three more unfavourable prenatal test results in the third, fourth and fifth pregnancy, the testee decided to make use of a PGD. This sixth pregnancy resulted in the birth of a child without the Huntington mutation.

In the group of carriers who did not mention reproductive decision-making as a motive for predictive testing for HD in the pretest period (N = 123) there were eight persons (7%) with one or more pregnancies after the communication of the predictive test result. One testee in this group had two pregnancies, the other seven each had one. Prenatal diagnosis was carried out in four of the nine pregnancies, resulting in three unfavourable results and one favourable result. All pregnancies with an unfavourable prenatal test result were terminated. Three testees had only one pregnancy, a pregnancy with a prenatal test. The testee with two further pregnancies had the first pregnancy tested and terminated after an unfavourable prenatal test result, and performed no prenatal test in the second pregnancy. Four testees had none of their pregnancies tested.

In the group of non-carriers reporting reproductive decision-making as a motive for predictive testing in the pretest period (N = 114) 56% of the testees had one or more pregnancies after the communication of the predictive test result. The total number of pregnancies after the predictive test in this group was 88. Forty-eight couples had one pregnancy, eight couples had two and eight couples had three further pregnancies.

In the group of non-carriers not reporting reproductive decision-making as a motive for predictive testing in the pretest period ($N = 157$) 12 testees had 1 pregnancy and 1 testee had 2 pregnancies after the predictive test. There were no miscarriages in this subgroup.

A comparison of the post predictive test reproductive history of carriers with and carriers without reproductive decision-making as a motive in the pretest period reveals a considerable difference in the number of testees who engage in one or more pregnancies: 18/57 (32%) in the former and 8/123 (7%) in the latter group. A comparison of the post predictive test reproduction of carriers and non-carriers with reproductive decision-making as a motive reveals a considerable difference: in the former group 18/57 (32%) engage in at least 1 pregnancy compared with 64/114 (56%) in the latter group. The fact that 19 of the 88 pregnancies (22%) of the non-carriers with family planning as a motive for predictive testing resulted in a miscarriage (eight testees had one miscarriage, four had two and one testee had three miscarriages), whereas there were no miscarriages in the non-carrier group without family planning as a motive in the pretest period is a finding without a clear explanation.

Reproductive history of carriers and non-carriers as a function of the presence or absence of family planning as a motive: data per genetic centre. Table 7 gives data per genetic centre regarding the post predictive test reproductive history of *carriers* as a function of the presence or absence of reproductive decision-making as a motive to apply for predictive testing in the pretest period. In the genetic centre at Leuven all carriers with family planning as a motive who had further pregnancies ($N = 7$) used prenatal testing. In Paris the proportion of carriers using prenatal testing was clearly lower. In Athens there was only one testee with further pregnancies and no prenatal diagnosis was performed. In the other centres the numbers of testees in this subgroup was too small. In the three centres with a sufficient number of testees to make a comparison between the subgroup with and without reproductive decision-making as a motive to apply for predictive testing, carriers without reproductive motives had a clearly lower number of pregnancies than carriers with reproductive decision-making as a motive for having a predictive test. The number of pregnancies in the former group is too small to compare the use of prenatal testing in both groups across the centres.

The same type of data for *non-carriers* is given in *Table 8*. The proportion of testees engaging in at least one pregnancy in the non-carrier group with family planning as a motive in the pretest period differs greatly from centre to centre. For the non-carriers without family planning as a motive the results are more similar across the centres. However, the small numbers are an impediment to drawing clear-cut conclusions.

For testees with family planning as a motive in the pretest period we compared per centre the likelihood of one or more subsequent pregnancies in the group of carriers of the Huntington mutation and in the group of non-carriers.

Table 7. Carriers' post predictive test reproduction as a function of the presence or absence of reproductive decision making as a motive for applying for predictive testing in the pretest period: data per centre

Carriers	Leuven (N = 28)	Cardiff (N = 23)	Paris (N = 38)	Leiden (N = 19)	Athens (N = 33)	Rome (N = 10)	Aberdeen (N = 29)	Total (N = 180)
Reproductive motive								
No. testees	16	2	18	3	16	2	0	57
No. testees with pregnancies	7	1	6	3	1	0	0	18
No. pregnancies	16	2	7	4	2	0	0	31
No. births (with PGD)	5 (1)	1	6	3	1	0	0	16
No. miscarriages	1	0	1	0	1	0	0	3
No. terminations	10	1	0	1	0	0	0	12
No. testees with prenatal tests	7	1	1	2	0	0	0	11
No. prenatal tests	14	2	1	3	0	0	0	20
No. favourable result	4	1	1	2	0	0	0	8
No. unfavourable result	10	1	0	1	0	0	0	12
No reproductive motive								
No. testees	12	21	20	16	17	8	29	123
No. testees with pregnancies	2	1	2	2	0	0	1	8
No. pregnancies	2	1	3	2	0	0	1	9
No. births	1	1	1	2	0	0	1	6
No. miscarriages	0	0	0	0	0	0	0	0
No. terminations	1	0	2	0	0	0	0	3
No. testees with prenatal tests	1	0	2	1	0	0	0	4
No. prenatal tests	1	0	2	1	0	0	0	4
No. favourable result	0	0	0	1	0	0	0	1
No. unfavourable result	1	0	2	0	0	0	0	3

Table 8. Non-carriers' post predictive test reproduction as a function of the presence or absence of reproductive decision making as a motive for applying for predictive testing in the pretest period: data per centre

Non-carriers	Leuven (N = 39)	Cardiff (N = 37)	Paris (N = 46)	Leiden (N = 39)	Athens (N = 59)	Rome (N = 19)	Aberdeen (N = 32)	Total (N = 271)
Reproductive motive								
No. testees	20	12	20	10	40	8	4	114
No. testees with pregnancies	11	1	9	7	30	3	3	64
No. pregnancies	14	1	10	11	45	3	4	88
No. births	13	1	5	10	33	3	3	68
No. miscarriages	1	0	4	1	12	0	1	19
No. terminations	0	0	1	0	0	0	0	1
No reproductive motive								
No. testees	19	25	26	29	19	11	28	157
No. testees with pregnancies	1	1	1	4	1	0	5	13
No. pregnancies	1	1	1	5	1	0	5	14
No. births	1	1	1	5	1	0	5	14
No. miscarriages	0	0	0	0	0	0	0	0
No. terminations	0	0	0	0	0	0	0	0

In Leuven and Paris the proportion engaging in at least one pregnancy is higher in the non-carrier group than in the carrier group, and the proportion is even higher in Athens and Rome. Here too the small numbers in some centres are an impediment to drawing conclusions.

Reproductive history for the subgroup of testees with a follow-up interval of at least three years and with reproductive decision-making as a major motive to apply for predictive testing.   In the previous paragraph the impact of the predictive test result on reproduction was evaluated by comparing the four subgroups (based on the variables 'carrier/non-carrier' and 'presence/absence of family planning motivation'). However, in this context, it is important to check whether the follow-up period is similar in the four subgroups. Unfortunately, this was not the case. The follow-up interval was significantly different in the four subgroups (*Table 9*). Analysis of variance revealed a significant main effect of the variables 'carrier status' ($F = 12.3$, $p < 0.001$) and 'presence/absence of reproductive decision-making as a motive to apply for predictive testing' ($F = 9.2$, $p < 0.01$) upon the follow-up interval. There was no significant interaction effect. Therefore, we focus on the reproductive history of the group of testees with a follow-up interval of three or more years and with reproductive decision-making as a major motive to apply for predictive testing (*Table 10*). This is indeed the most appropriate group to evaluate the effect of the predictive test result on reproduction. This group consists of 96 testees, 40% carriers and 60% non-carriers. In the group of carriers ($N = 38$) there were 15 persons (39%) with pregnancies after the predictive test. The total number of pregnancies in these 15 persons was 25. These pregnancies resulted in 14 births, 3 miscarriages and 8 terminations. Eight of the fifteen testees had one or more prenatal tests. In this group there were 15 prenatal tests performed, resulting in 7 favourable and 8 unfavourable results. In the group of non-carriers 69% had further pregnancies. The 58 pregnancies in this group resulted in 43 births, 14 miscarriages and 1 termination (for reasons other than HD).

The above results in this particular subgroup, which is most adequate for this type of evaluation, clearly show a definite impact of the predictive test result on reproductive decision-making. In the carrier group the percentage of testees engaging in one or more pregnancies (69%) is indeed much higher than in the non-carrier group (39%). Moreover, a completely different type of analysis, namely an analysis of covariance testing the effect of the predictive test result upon having or not having further pregnancies after the predictive test, keeping age at the time of

Table 9. Mean follow-up interval (in months) as a function of carrier status and the presence or absence of family planning motives in the pretest period

	Carrier ($N = 180$)	Non-carrier ($N = 271$)
Family planning is a motive	45 (SD, 24)	39 (SD, 26)
Family planning is not a motive	40 (SD, 23)	29 (SD, 24)

Table 10. Post predictive test reproduction in the subgroup with at least 3 years follow-up with family planning as a motive in the pretest period

	Carriers (N = 38)	Non-carriers (N = 58)	Total (N = 96)
No. testees without pregnancies	23 (61%)	18 (31%)	41 (43%)
No. testees with pregnancies	15 (39%)	40 (69%)	55 (57%)
No. pregnancies	25	58	83
No. births	14	43	57
No. miscarriages	3	14	17
No. terminations	8	1	9
No. testees with prenatal tests	8		8
No. prenatal tests	15		15
No. favourable	7		7
No. unfavourable	8		8

the predictive test and the number of pregnancies before the predictive test under control, confirmed that the predictive test result had a significant effect upon having further pregnancies after the predictive test ($F = 8.46$; $p < 0.01$).

Special issues in evaluating the impact of the predictive test result on subsequent reproduction: How to deal with testees who were pregnant at the time of the communication of the predictive test result?

For couples with a pregnancy at the time of the communication of the predictive test result the pregnancy was considered as a pregnancy in the pretest period, no matter what the outcome of the pregnancy (birth, miscarriage or termination). As a consequence, all these pregnancies were integrated in the data regarding reproductive history before predictive testing (although the outcome of the pregnancy may only be visible after the communication of the test result). There were 14 couples with a pregnancy at the time of the communication of the predictive test result (3.5% of the total group of testees). In four of the couples one of the partners was revealed to be a carrier (29%), in the other couples the testee was revealed to be a non-carrier. In half of the couples the mother belonged to a Huntington family, in the other half the father.

The onset of the disease in some of the carriers may play a part in the reproductive history after predictive testing. Because of their age at the time of predictive testing and depending on the length of the follow-up interval, it is probable that some carriers already presented symptoms of HD at the time of the last follow-up contact. For some carriers, data were available on the onset of the disease, for others there was 'vague' information on the presence or absence of symptoms, for others there is no information at all. In 21% of the cases it is unknown or uncertain whether the carrier (already) had any symptoms of HD. For 66% there was no evidence at all for any symptoms during the most recent follow-up contact. The last 13% of the carriers had symptoms either mentioned by themselves during the follow-up contacts, either mentioned by the professional, or both. The available data were not sufficiently detailed to allow any conclusion on the consequences of the 'awareness of symptoms' for the reproductive behaviour in the former group.

How complete was the family at the time of the last follow-up contact? Forty-three per cent of the testees considered their family to be complete at the time of the last follow-up contact, whereas 27% considered it incomplete at that time. Fourteen per cent were still undecided about having (additional) pregnancies and for 16% of the testees this information was unknown or unavailable. In the group of carriers for whom information is available 59% considered their family complete, 29% incomplete and 12% were undecided. In the group of non-carriers for whom information is available 46% considered their family complete, 34% incomplete and 20% were undecided.

What about the reproductive history of testees with an intermediate allele? In the total group of testees ($N = 453$) there were two testees with an intermediate allele. The first person with an intermediate allele was tested in 1993. This testee was a female, aged 34 years. She was in a stable relationship and had one child (born in 1985) and a miscarriage (occurred in 1988) before the predictive test. She took the predictive test for reason of certainty and informing her child. The last contact occurred in 1999. She had no pregnancies after predictive testing and at the time of the last contact she expressed that her family was complete. The second testee with an intermediate allele was tested in 1996. It was a woman aged 29 years with a stable relationship. She had one child before the predictive test. She applied for a predictive test for family planning reasons and for informing her child. In 1999 she made an appointment for a counselling session to obtain information about PGD because she wanted a second child. She and her partner had objections against abortion. There was no later follow-up contact. This is just a description of the 'facts'. In this type of study it is unfortunately not possible to assess the exact impact on reproductive decision-making of an 'intermediate' allele compared with an unfavourable test result consisting of a number of repeats in the common range for HD. This can only be done by in-depth interviews in well-elaborated case presentations.

3. Discussion

In most countries where the predictive test is available, it is estimated that fewer than one-fifth of the persons at risk for HD have had a predictive test. The motivation to have a predictive test for this currently untreatable late-onset disease is very complex and moreover it is a mixture of conscious and unconscious motives. The most frequently mentioned reason to apply for predictive testing is 'having certainty'. Family planning is also a reason that is frequently mentioned by applicants at reproductive age, either in combination with 'having certainty' or as a single reason. In the present European collaborative study 'reproductive decision-making' was mentioned as an important reason by 38% of the testees.

When a predictive test applicant mentions 'family planning' as a motive for predictive testing in the pretest period this may have a completely different meaning from one applicant to the other. A first group of persons with a desire for children 'does not want to transmit the Huntington mutation to the next generation'. When they develop scenarios about reproductive decision-making should the predictive test reveal that they are a carrier, they may have in mind one of the following alternatives: not having children, having pregnancies with prenatal diagnosis or making use of IVF and PGD. The latter option is very recent and is available in only a few centres in the world (Chapter 7). Two other options, artificial insemination with donor sperm or IVF with egg cell donation are considered extremely rarely, even more rarely after the availability of predictive and prenatal DNA testing. Adoption is a third option and seems very rarely chosen. A second group does not want to have children, should they carry the mutation, because they 'do not want to confront their children with a parent who may become affected during their children's childhood or adolescence'. This conviction may be induced by negative experiences with the disease of their affected parent, in particular in situations in which the psychiatric problems of the parent had a strong impact on their own life and/or on their siblings' life during childhood or adolescence. There may of course be an overlap between the two groups. Moreover, the weight given to each of the two aspects (transmission of the mutation and impact of an affected parent on the children's education and life) may differ from one couple to another and also between the two members of the same couple or within the same person from one period to another. A third group may need a predictive test result 'for planning the exact number of children or for timing the birth of their children' e.g. postpone children in case of a favourable predictive test result (because they have a subjective feeling of 'more time') and having children as soon as possible in the case of an unfavourable predictive test result (because of a subjective feeling of time pressure). We should be very well aware of the fact that the length of the follow-up interval of this type of studies becomes more important because of the last group of testees: a longer follow-up interval may increase the difference in reproduction between carriers and non-carriers. This is also the reason why the type of evaluation in the present study should be repeated with a follow-up interval of at least 10 years.

During the pretest counselling sessions the complexity of the motive 'family planning' and its situation-specific character is often illustrated (see also Chapters 2 and 8). For a discussion of the family perspective on this issue we refer to Watkin and Varkevisser (Chapter 10). Depending on the testees' and their partner's moral and/or religious convictions or values some reproductive options may be excluded. For a discussion of the ethical aspects of some reproductive options and for the legal aspects related to pregnancy termination, including the differences in law from one country to the other we refer respectively to Chapters 6 and 9. Although this is less relevant in a study evaluating the impact of the predictive test result on subsequent reproduction, it is nevertheless important to draw the attention on the importance of adequate counselling when a couple applies for exclusion testing. It is important to discuss all implications of not wanting to transmit the Huntington mutation and at the same time not wanting to know their own carrier status. Prenatal exclusion testing is discussed in several chapters in this book.

The European collaborative study has directly addressed the question whether a predictive test result for HD has an effect on subsequent reproduction. To answer this question the reproduction of carriers and non-carriers of the Huntington mutation, who were not older than 45 years, was compared. A unique characteristic of this study is that this evaluation is carried out in persons of reproductive age who had a predictive test following the identification of the Huntington gene and who were counselled in one of the participating genetic centres using a well-defined pretest and post-test counselling approach. Moreover data about the motives for applying for predictive testing as reported in the pretest period were available in the files. Thanks to the European collaboration, data were collected for a group of 180 carriers and 271 non-carriers who meet the above criteria and who received a predictive test result in the period 1993–1998 in Aberdeen, Athens, Cardiff, Leiden, Leuven, Paris and Rome. The mean age of the total study group was 31.5 years and for about half of the group the follow-up interval was 3 years or more.

The European collaborative study clearly revealed a measurable impact of the predictive test result on subsequent reproduction: 14% of the total group of carriers had one or more subsequent pregnancies compared with 28% of the total group of non-carriers. A prenatal test was carried out in about two-thirds of the pregnancies in the carrier group. One couple had chosen IVF and PGD, resulting in the birth of a child before the last follow-up contact. During the post-test counselling sessions a very small number of couples in the carrier group expressed plans to make use of PGD in the future. A more refined analysis was performed in the subgroup that is most adequate for this type of evaluation study, namely the group who reported 'family planning' as a motive to apply for predictive testing in the pretest period and with a follow-up interval of at least 3 years. In this subgroup the effect was more pronounced: 39% of the carriers of the Huntington mutation had subsequent pregnancies compared with 69% of the non-carriers. Notwithstanding a desire for children or the presence of 'family planning' as one of the major reasons to apply for predictive testing, the majority of carriers had no subsequent pregnancy. It can be hypothesized that the difference between carriers and non-carriers might even have become more pronounced should we have used a longer follow-up interval (cf. the first part of this discussion concerning the meaning of the motive 'family planning'). A prenatal test was carried out in slightly fewer than two-thirds of the pregnancies in the carrier group. Of course the family may not yet be complete for part of the group. The relatively small numbers in the subgroup that is optimal for this type of analysis did not allow drawing clear-cut conclusions regarding differences between centres.

It is clear from the above findings that predictive DNA testing helps some couples to fulfil their desire to have children without risk of transmitting the mutation. Some carriers for whom family planning was initially a motive for applying for predictive testing and who had the intention, in the pretest period, of avoiding the risk of transmitting the disease, seem to have changed their minds after they were revealed to be carriers of the Huntington mutation. Intentions and behaviour are not always the same, as has already been shown in the context of predictive and prenatal testing and in many other situations.

In considering all these findings it is important to keep in mind that only a minority of persons at risk for HD make use of predictive testing and prenatal testing. Nevertheless, although systematic research on the non-tested group is lacking, all professionals confronted with families with HD have experienced in practice that reproductive decision-making in this situation of increased genetic risk usually is and remains a difficult dilemma. It is also clear that the final decision is not always the result of well-structured or rational decision-making, as is the case for many other important life decisions. Decision difficulties and ambivalence are also illustrated by the fact that some applicants for predictive testing have become pregnant in the months or weeks preceding the communication of the predictive test result (Decruyenaere *et al.*, 1996). It is clear that a wide variety of emotional factors, transgenerational loyalties and so far unknown issues (including counselling style even within a standardized test protocol?) play a part in reproductive decision-making in a situation of increased genetic risk for late-onset disease. To date there is not much evidence in families with HD in Europe that couples 'take the risk' because of an optimistic hope for cure. This seems different from the situation in Canada (Hayden, 2001). Whatever option is chosen by a couple at increased risk of transmitting the Huntingon mutation, it is of the utmost importance that professionals fully respect and support the couple in implementing this decision.

Acknowledgements

The authors explicitly acknowledge the contribution of the many persons in the participating genetic centres without whom the present study would have been impossible. In Leuven (Belgium): Dr M. Decruyenaere, Mrs T. Cloostermans, Mrs A. Boogaerts, Professor Dr G. Matthijs and Professor Dr J.-P. Fryns. In Cardiff (UK): Dr R. Harper and Mrs R. Glew. In Leiden (The Netherlands): Dr J.A. Maat-Kievit, Professor dr M.H. Breuning, Dr M. Losekoot, Professor Dr B. Bakker and Mrs M.N. Ané. In Paris (France): Professor Dr Josué Feingold, Mrs Marcela Garguilo, Mrs Tecla Capecchi, Dr Khadija Lahlou. In Rome (Italy): Dr M. Frontali. In Athens (Greece): Professor C. Papageorgiou, Professor M.Dalakas, Professor D.Vassilopoulos, Dr C. Voumvourakis, Dr M. Panas, Mrs S. Pomoni (Department of Neurology, University of Athens). Last, but not least, the authors would like to express special gratitude to Mrs N. Opdekamp for secretarial assistance during the study and during the preparation of this chapter.

References

Adam, S., Wiggins, S., Whyte, P., et al (1993) Five year study of prenatal testing for Huntington's disease: demand, attitudes and psychological assessment. *J. Med. Genet.* **30:** 549–556.

Craufurd, D., Dodge, A., Kerzin-Storrar, L. and Harris, R. (1989) Uptake of presymptomatic predictive testing for Huntington's disease (letter). *Lancet*; **2:** 603–605.

Decruyenaere, M., Evers-Kiebooms, G., Boogaerts, A., Cassiman, J.J., Cloostermans, T., Demyttenaere, K., Dom, R., Fryns, J.-P. and Van den Berghe H. (1996) Prediction of psychological functioning one year after the predictive test for Huntington's disease and impact of the test result on reproductive decision-making. *J. Med. Genet.* 33: 737–743.

Decruyenaere, M., Evers-Kiebooms, G., Boogaerts, A., Cassiman, J.J., Cloostermans, T., Demyttenaere, K., Dom, R., Fryns, J.-P. and Van den Berghe, H. (1997) Non participation in predictive testing for Huntington's disease: individual decision-making, personality and avoidment behaviour in the family. *Eur. J. Hum. Genet.* 5: 351–363.

Evers-Kiebooms, G. (1997) Recent evolutions in prenatal testing for Huntington's disease. Presentation during the 17th International Meeting of the World Federation of Neurology Research Group on Huntington's Disease, Sydney, August

Evers-Kiebooms, G., Fryns, J.P., Demyttenaere, K., Decruyenaere, M., Boogaerts, A., Cloostermans, T., Cassiman, J.-J., Dom, R. and Van den Berghe, H. (1996) Predictive and preimplantation genetic testing for Huntington's disease and other late-onset dominant disorders: not in conflict but complementary (letter). *Clin. Genet.* 50: 275–276.

Evers-Kiebooms, G., Nys, K., Harper, P., Zoeteweij, M., Dürr, A., Jacopini, G., Yapijakis, C. and Simpson, S. (2002) Predictive DNA-testing for Huntington's disease and reproductive decision-making: a European collaborative study *Eur. J. Hum. Genet.* 10: 167–176.

Evers-Kiebooms, G., Welkenhuysen, M., Claes, E. , Decruyenaere, M. and Denayer, L. (2000) The psychological complexity of predictive testing for late onset neurogenetic diseases and hereditary cancers. *Soc. Sci. Med.* 51: 831–841.

Harper, P. (1996) *Huntington's Disease.* Saunders, London.

Harper, P., Lim, C. and Craufurd, D. (2000) Ten years of presymptomatic testing for Huntington's disease: the experience of the U.K. Huntington's Disease Prediction Consortium. *J. Med. Genet.* 37: 567–571.

Hayden, M.R. (2001) Predictive testing for Huntington disease – 15 years later. Presentation during the International Congress of Human Genetics in Vienna, 15 May.

Hayden, M.R., Bloch, M. and Wiggins, S. (1995) Psychological effects of predictive testing for Huntington's disease. *Behav. Neurol. Mov. Disord.* 65: 201–210.

Huntington's Disease Collaborative Research Group. (1993) A novel gene containing a trinucleotide repeat that is expanded and unstable on Huntington's disease chromosomes. *Cell* 72: 971–983.

International Huntington Association and World Federation of Neurology (1994) Guidelines for the molecular genetics predictive test in Huntington's disease. *Neurology* 44: 1533–1536.

Lippman-Hand, A. and Fraser, F.C. (1979) Genetic counselling – the postcounselling period: II. Making reproductive choices. *Am. J. Med. Genet.* 4: 73–87.

Maat-Kievit, A., Vegter-van der Vlis, M., Zoeteweij, M., Losekoot, M., van Haeringen, A., Kanhai, H. and Roos, R. (1999) Experience in prenatal testing for Huntington's disease in the Netherlands: procedures, results and guidelines (1987–1997). *Prenat. Diagn.* 19: 450–457.

Quaid, K.A. and Morris, M. (1993) M. Reluctance to undergo predictive testing: the case of Huntington disease. *Am. J. Med.* 45: 41–45.

Schulman, J.D., Black, S.H., Handyside, A. and Nance, W.E. (1996) Preimplantation genetic testing for Huntington's disease and certain other dominantly inherited disorders. *Clin. Genet.* 49: 57–58.

Simpson, S., Zoeteweij, M., Nys, K., Harper, P., Dürr, A., Jacopini, G., Yapijakis, C. and Evers-Kiebooms, G. Prenatal testing for Huntington's disease: A European collaborative study (submitted).

Tolmie, J.L., Davidson, H.R., May, H.M., McIntosh, K., Paterson, J.S. and Smith, B. (1995) The prenatal exclusion test for Huntington's disease: experience in the west of Scotland, 1986–1993. *J. Med. Genet.* 32: 97–101.

Tyler, A., Ball, D. and Craufurd, D. (1992) Presymptomatic testing for Huntington's disease in the United Kingdom. *Br. Med. J.* 304: 1593–1596.

Tyler, A., Quarrell, O., Lazarou, L.P., Meredith, A.L. and Harper, P.S. (1990) Exclusion testing in pregnancy for Huntington's disease. *J. Med. Genet.* 27: 488–495.

Van der Steenstraten, I., Tibben, A., Roos, R.A., Van de Kamp, J.J. and Niermeijer, M.F. (1994) Predictive testing for Huntington disease: nonparticipants compared with participants in the Dutch program. *Am. J. Hum. Genet.* **55:** 618–625.

5

Predictive and prenatal testing for Huntington's disease in Greece, Germany, Austria, Switzerland and Denmark

Christos Yapijakis, Franco Laccone and Sven Asger Sørensen

1. Introduction

The assignment of the Huntington's disease (HD) gene to chromosome 4 by Gusella *et al.* in 1983 made it possible to perform presymptomatic and prenatal diagnostic tests by linkage analysis. Huntington's disease was the first severe, autosomal dominantly inherited disorder with late onset for which these diagnostic possibilities became available. This potential aroused a worldwide discussion among scientists, physicians and lay persons on the ethical and psychosocial consequences of the introduction of such procedures. These discussions resulted in the guidelines of the International Huntington Association and World Federation of Neurology Research Group on Huntington's Chorea (1990) which were revised in 1994, after the positional cloning of the huntingtin gene (Huntington Disease Collaborative Research Group, 1993).

Predictive and prenatal testing for HD were initiated in the USA, UK and Canada as early as 1987 (Farrer *et al.*, 1988; Harper *et al.*, 1990; Hayden *et al.*, 1987; Quarrell *et al.*, 1987). By 1989 HD testing was available in 13 countries, including Greece, Germany, Switzerland and Denmark. A worldwide survey, which was published after the cloning of the responsible mutant gene (World Federation of Neurology Research Group on Huntington's Chorea, 1993),

Prenatal Testing for Late-Onset Neurogenetic Diseases, edited by G. Evers-Kiebooms, M. W. Zoeteweij and P. S. Harper

reported that a total of 1479 completed predictive tests had been performed in 19 countries using RFLP analysis. According to the same survey, the first three countries (ranked by number of tests performed) were UK, Canada and USA, whereas Greece, Switzerland, Denmark and Germany were 7th, 9th, 10th and 14th, respectively. Ranked by number of tests performed per centre, the first three countries were The Netherlands, Greece and Denmark, all of which had a national centralized testing facility in Leiden, Athens and Copenhagen, respectively.

Identification of an expanded $(CAG)_n$ repeat in the huntingtin gene as the primary cause of HD (Huntington Disease Collaborative Research Group, 1993) prompted direct molecular analysis of affected and at-risk individuals in several countries, including Germany, Denmark and Greece (Norremolle *et al.*, 1993; Yapijakis *et al.*, 1995; Zuhlke *et al.*, 1993). The direct test solved many of the previous problems with the linkage analysis approach, such as availability of informative family members, and confidentiality or collaboration among relatives. However, an initially increased demand for predictive and prenatal testing reached a plateau in the following years, since then in fact only a small percentage of at-risk individuals have desired to know their status, in light of an as yet elusive therapy.

In this chapter, the decade-long experience of five European countries regarding presymptomatic and prenatal testing for HD is presented (summarized in *Table 1*). In Denmark and Greece a unique national public centre has undertaken the performance of the tests. In Germany, Austria and Switzerland there are 17 public and 6 private laboratories, all of which belong to a consortium for HD testing in German-speaking populations.

2. Greece

2.1 Presymptomatic and prenatal testing for Huntington's disease: the Greek experience

The incidence of HD in Greece is estimated to be similar to that in other European countries, i.e. about 1 patient in 10 000 individuals. Since the Greek population is roughly 10 600 000, it follows that there are probably about 1000 HD patients and, according to Conneally (1984), at least three times as many individuals at risk (3000) in Greece.

Table 1. Predictive and prenatal testing for Huntington's disease in five European countries

	Predictive tests		Prenatal tests	
	First test	Total number	First test	Total number
Denmark	1989	399	1991	40
Greece	1989	205	1991	3
Germany	1989	886	1993	23
Switzerland	1987	89	1995	1
Austria	1993	17	–	0

Diagnostic molecular testing for HD was established relatively early in Greece (by 1989). Presymptomatic diagnostic testing has been offered by a unique genetic centre at the University of Athens Medical School, initially using linkage analysis (1989–1992) and since 1993 by mutation detection (Yapijakis *et al.*, 1991, 1995). Predictive testing has been performed according to the guidelines of the International Huntington Association and World Federation of Neurology Group on Huntington's Chorea (1990, 1994a, 1994b). Huntington's disease patients and their families have been referred from various parts of Greece, mainly from university departments of neurology. The number of predictive tests performed over the decade is 205, accounting for 6.8% of the putatively existing individuals at risk. In addition, to date, the same genetic centre has performed only three prenatal tests, the first as early as 1991 (Yapijakis *et al.*, 1993). In a country like Greece, where other prenatal diagnostic tests have been performed routinely for more than two decades, the observed extremely low amount of prenatal versus presymptomatic testing is surprising. As the relevant data from Greece are presented in Chapters 3 and 4 as part of the European collaborative study, the following text attempts to find possible explanations for the low uptake of predictive and prenatal tests for HD in this country.

2.2 Prenatal testing for genetic disorders in Greece

Prenatal testing for genetic or congenital disorders has a long history in Greece and is widely accepted by society as a preventive practice. Depending on the nature of the tested disorder, a cytogenetic, biochemical or molecular approach may be used.

Cytogenetic testing was initiated as early as 1976 for the prenatal diagnosis of chromosomal abnormalities and is currently performed in more than six public and three private genetic centres in Greece (Metaxotou *et al.*, 1997). It is estimated that karyotype examination is performed in >80% of high-risk pregnancies. Major indications for prenatal testing include advanced maternal age (>35 years), increased risk for chromosomal disorders because of a triple hormone test at week 16 with/without an abnormal US nuchal translucency, an inherited chromosomal disorder. About 7000 prenatal tests are performed annually, accounting for >7% of the total number of pregnancies (Metaxotou, personal communication). Of these 7000 prenatal cytogenetic tests, most are performed on amniotic fluid samples (about 5000), whereas the rest involve chorionic villi (about 1500) and fetal blood samples (about 500).

Biochemical prenatal testing is less common in Greece, with the exception of the widely used indicative triple hormone test at week 16 of gestation (chorionic gonadotropin, free estradiol and α-fetal protein). It is estimated that >70% of pregnant women under 35 years of age have this test annually, in order to estimate their fetus' risk for a chromosomal disorder.

However, molecular prenatal testing has a tradition of 10–20 years, with about 15 inherited disorders tested in a routine manner. Common recessive disorders, such as β-thalassaemia and cystic fibrosis, are widely tested for (Kanavakis *et al.*, 1997; Kollia *et al.*, 1992; Loukopoulos *et al.*, 1985, 1990;

Tzetis *et al.*, 1997). In particular, β-thalassaemia is very common in the Greek population with carriers accounting for 5–10% of the population in some regions. The Greek programme of molecular testing for β-thalassaemia, which includes carrier detection and prenatal diagnosis, has been so successful that it represents an internationally unparalleled paradigm of eradication of a common genetic disorder through a prevention strategy, in addition to the equivalent one in Cyprus (Angastiniotis *et al.*, 1988). The respective preventive programmes for β-thalassaemia in Greece and Cyprus have a prevention rate of new cases of 98.5 and 99.8% respectively. Massive carrier detection has been available following informative consent since 1983 in Greece, and has been obligatory for newlywed couples since 1987 in Cyprus.

2.3 Molecular prenatal testing in Greece: the paradigms of thalassaemia and Huntington's disease

Careful comparison of the highly successful preventive programme for thalassaemia and the extremely low uptake of the preventive programme for HD may reveal the different parameters that have influenced the diverse outcome of these projects. Obviously, the two disorders are not completely comparable, because they differ in frequency of mutation carriers, mode of inheritance, age of onset and the best prevention strategy (carrier detection in thalassaemia versus presymptomatic diagnosis in HD). However, both share some characteristics, including a severe and eventually lethal symptomatology, the need for technically accurate molecular testing and arising psychosocial issues.

Social parameters regarding prenatal testing are mostly common for both HD and thalassaemia. In Greek society there is a general acceptance of prenatal testing for severe disorders, mainly because of the long-standing and widely publicized programmes against chromosomal disorders and thalassaemia (Mavrou *et al.*, 1998). As a rule, the State has set the legal stage for 'appropriate' prenatal testing and tried to promote high-quality public services in the past two decades. Nevertheless, there are still things to be done, namely the establishment of the long-awaited specialty of medical genetics and the rational coordination of available public genetic centres, which are administered by the Ministry of Health. The Orthodox Christian Church of Greece has assumed a practically neutral position towards prenatal testing, and has managed to both officially consider it as 'an act of murder in the eyes of God' and at the same time to maintain a rather inactive posture to such a widely accepted practice. As a result, the anti-abortion movement is almost non-existent in Greece.

Regarding the health specialists involved in prenatal testing for both thalassaemia and HD, they fall into two categories, namely the genetic centres and the referring doctors. There are four public centres involved in prenatal testing for thalassaemia with 10–20 years' experience, and a unique one for HD with 10 years' experience. The technical quality of the offered molecular services is of a similar high standard in all centres, but genetic counselling is understandably practised in more depth at the HD centre. So far, no parameter has appeared to be obviously different accounting for the discrepancy in numbers of the prenatal testing uptake for the two disorders.

Last, but not least, the referring doctors are the key mediators who first inform the at-risk part of the Greek population about prenatal testing and possibly refer them to the appropriate centre. For thalassaemia, the referring doctors may be a variety of specialists, including (mainly) obstetricians, geneticists, haematologists and paediatricians. In contrast, for HD, the referring doctors are almost always neurologists and rarely geneticists. Surprisingly, referring doctors constitute a major difference between the paradigms of β-thalassaemia and HD.

2.4 Attitudes of Greek neurologists towards genetic testing for Huntington's disease

In order to assess the major characteristics of Greek neurologists regarding their attitudes on HD genetic testing and genetic counselling, data from an opinion survey were analysed (Yapijakis *et al.*, 1998). Most Greek neurologists regard HD as a devastating, chronic and progressive neurodegenerative disorder, for which a really effective treatment does not yet exist. However, predictive genetic testing and genetic counselling seem to them untrustworthy, unknown, unnecessary and likely to do more harm than good. The lack of an officially recognized specialty of medical genetics in Greece leads to the existing limited acceptance of new scientific developments and the deficient management of at-risk individuals and families.

Greek university neurologists, in particular, tend to be more knowledgeable about molecular genetics, but they think that it is useful mainly for establishing a clinical diagnosis or for research. They consider presymptomatic or prenatal testing unjustified, and genetic counselling not fully necessary. For example, there is one professor of neurology who uses molecular techniques in his research on HD, but is not interested in establishing predictive/prenatal testing in his centre.

Therefore, it is not surprising that very few neurologists in Greece inform the patients' relatives about the possibility of a predictive test. Even if asked, most advise at-risk individuals to abstain from having children, as a prevention strategy. The fact that there are extremely few general practitioners and neurogeneticists in Greece and there is no layman's association for HD renders neurologists as a practically unique source of information and advice for the HD families.

2.5 Future prospects

The Greek state is planning to establish a national system of medical genetic services for all interested individuals and families in the country, as part of the National Health System (ESY). The successful preventive programme for thalassaemia may be used as a model system. There is currently a committee of reknowned geneticists, working under the auspices of the Ministry of Health, which is expected to propose the guidelines for training and qualification of the to-be-established specialties of medical genetics (including clinical genetics and laboratory genetics). Existing centres in the country will serve as training and reference centres. In addition, the specialty of neurology has recently started to include 6 months of training in neurogenetics.

3. Germany, Austria and Switzerland

3.1 Brief history

After the cloning of the HD gene in 1993, a consortium of clinicians, geneticists, patient support groups and laboratories offering molecular testing for HD from Germany, Switzerland and Austria was founded. The aim of this consortium was to develop an interdisciplinary approach to the new possibilities offered by molecular testing and to discuss the medical, ethical, legal and technical issues connected to molecular testing and other present topics at an annual meeting.

One of the first decisions adopted by the consortium was the recommendation to carry out both the presymptomatic and diagnostic tests according to the international guidelines for the molecular diagnosis of HD (International Huntington Association and World Federation of Neurology Research Group on Huntington's Chorea, 1994a, 1994b). Furthermore, it was possible to begin quality control of the genotyping and to develop standards for the precise determination of the CAG repeat number (Laccone, unpublished data). The number of laboratories offering prenatal and presymptomatic testing increased very rapidly after 1998 and currently consists of 23 laboratories, 6 of which are private. The data collected by the consortium regarding the presymptomatic and prenatal diagnosis carried out in these three countries from 1993 to 1997 have been retrospectively collected and evaluated (Laccone *et al.*, 1999). The data reported here concern only direct testing for HD.

3.2 Presymptomatic testing for Huntington's disease in Germany, Austria and Switzerland

Twelve laboratories of the Consortium for DNA Analysis of HD provided data on age and gender for each individual requesting a presymptomatic test. The *a priori* risk was not assessed because of the lack of comprehensive data for all persons at risk evaluated in this study. Altogether 992 persons at risk required a presymptomatic test (Germany 886, Switzerland 89 and Austria 17). Three hundred and seventy individuals have been found to be carriers of an expanded allele (>39 CAG repeats) and these persons have therefore been considered to be at high risk for developing HD. Fifty-two have an allele of 27–35 CAG repeats (normal mutable allele). Thirty individuals have been found to have alleles of 36–39 repeats (alleles of reduced penetrance). Five hundred and forty individuals have two alleles in the non-expanded range (27 CAG repeats). The mean age of the tested group was 34.8 years. However, 50% of the population at risk requested molecular testing at between 23 and 33 years of age with a clear predominance of women (ratio, 1.37). The women-to-men ratio in the remaining individuals at risk was 1.30. The uptake of the tests from 1993 to 1997 is shown in *Figure 1*.

Because the combined population of the three countries is about 100 million and considering the incidence of HD to be 1 in 10 000, there is an estimated HD patient population of about 10 000. It has been calculated (Conneally,

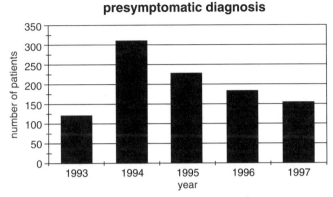

Figure 1. Annual uptake of the presymptomatic tests in Germany, Austria and Switzerland.

1984) that there should be at least three persons at risk per affected individual. The calculated at-risk population would therefore be about 30 000.

Following cloning of the gene a dramatic increase in the number of requests for testing was foreseen by several authors. These expectations were based principally on studies about attitudes towards presymptomatic diagnosis of HD which were carried out before direct testing was possible. In a survey on the attitudes of the German population towards presymptomatic testing for HD, 67% of persons at risk said that they would consider a presymptomatic test and 45% would require a prenatal test (Kreuz, 1996). The predicted demand for direct presymptomatic testing was, however, not apparent. In fact, fewer than 3% of the eligible population in our countries requested a test. This discrepancy between attitudes before and after the discovery that a single mutation accounts for HD is not specific for German-speaking countries but has been observed worldwide. However, it seems that in Germany, Switzerland and Austria the number of requests is much lower than in other European countries.

Two recently published papers from The Netherlands and the UK allow comparison of the uptake of predictive testing for HD in these countries with our data (Harper *et al.*, 2000; Maat-Kievit *et al.*, 2000). Germany, Austria, Switzerland, the UK and The Netherlands are, to a large extent, comparable in terms of health care, genetic counselling facilities, free accessibility to these structures and socio-economic profile. The absolute number of tests performed

Table 2. Presymptomatic and prenatal tests in the German-speaking countries, in the UK and in The Netherlands

	Germany, Austria, Switzerland	United Kingdom	The Netherlands
Presymptomatic	992	2502	752*
Prenatal	24	111	41
Population	96 million	60 million	16 million

*Also includes data from indirect testing from 1987 to 1993.

Table 3. Projection of the hypothetical uptake of the presymptomatic and prenatal tests in The Netherlands and in the UK supposing an equal population like the total one of the German-speaking countries

	Germany, Austria, Switzerland	United Kingdom	The Netherlands
Presymptomatic	992	4003	4512
Prenatal	24	178	246
Population	96 million	96 million	96 million

is reported in *Table 2*. A projection regarding the number of tests requested if the UK and The Netherlands would have a population of 96 million inhabitants equal to the combined population of Germany, Austria and Switzerland, is given in *Table 3*. Although the comparison in such a hypothetical situation might be influenced by several factors and therefore biased, the differences are very striking and highly significant. The reasons for the very low interest of the German-speaking populations in the predictive test of HD are not very clear and have not been investigated. Without doubt, however, experiences during the Nazi regime may play an important role in this respect. It is also possible that tragic events, such as murders, the sterilization of HD patients and other types of crimes perpetrated by the Nazis, have so deeply scared HD families, that they still have an unconscious fear of being discriminated against and hurt. Complementary to this is the lack of a central roster such as the one in The Netherlands, a fact which makes very difficult to ascertain the number of persons at risk and to inform them about the existence of presymptomatic molecular genetic testing.

Independent of the specifically German features, there are objective reasons for the worldwide low uptake of presymptomatic and prenatal diagnosis for HD. Huntington's disease is a late-onset disease and this has allowed persons at risk to hope for the development of a therapy in the near future. At the same time, the absence of an efficient therapy led the vast majority of individuals at risk to consider the presymptomatic test as useless. During the last 3 years we have observed no increase in the number of requests for presymptomatic testing in our populations. However, because of the increased numbers of laboratories carrying out molecular testing this steady trend might be biased. Nevertheless, there is general agreement that the number of requests for presymptomatic testing would increase rapidly in case of the availability of a therapy able to mitigate the course of the disease.

3.3 Prenatal testing for Huntington's disease in Germany, Austria and Switzerland

Requests for prenatal testing have been extremely rare. Prenatal testing has been performed in 24 cases. A summary of the requests and their outcomes are shown in *Table 4*. One woman at risk requested a prenatal diagnosis in three subsequent pregnancies. The first prenatal diagnosis found her to be a carrier of a fetus having an expanded allele. Altogether six fetuses had an expanded

Table 4. Prenatal tests in Germany and Switzerland

Features	Number/per cent
50% risk for the fetus	15
25% risk for the fetus	9
Average *a priori* risk	40%
Expected fetuses with expanded alleles	9
Observed fetuses with expanded alleles	6
Terminations	2

allele. Two pregnancies have been terminated, notably in the woman requesting three prenatal diagnoses. One pregnancy was continued. No further information was available for the remaining three pregnancies. Although there are insufficient data about the total number of pregnancies in couples at risk, prenatal diagnosis is not considered a realistic reproductive choice for HD families, at least in German-speaking countries.

4. Denmark

4.1 Predictive testing for Huntington's disease in Denmark

In 1989, a protocol for predictive tests and prenatal investigations for HD was approved by the Danish Scientific Committee of Ethics and the diagnostic procedures were offered to persons at risk for HD. Since the introduction of presymptomatic and prenatal investigations in Denmark, testing has been centralized at the Department of Medical Genetics in Copenhagen where the Danish Huntington Register is located. Blood samples and DNA from all affected HD patients have been collected systematically since 1983. Thus, DNA from affected grandparents is available in most cases for the exclusion test. Up to the first half of 2001, a total of 399 presymptomatic tests had been performed.

The first request for a prenatal investigation was in 1991. Here we present the results of 10 years of prenatal investigations for HD in Denmark.

4.2 Prenatal testing for Huntington's disease in Denmark: a decade of data

During the period 1991–2000, 40 prenatal tests in 30 couples were performed in Denmark (*Table 5*). This represents only a small fraction of the pregnancies

Table 5. Number of prenatal investigations for Huntington's disease in 30 couples in Denmark (1991–2000)

	Number of prenatal investigations					
	1	2	3	4	5	Total
No. females	11	1	–	–	–	12
No. males	14	1	2	–	1	18
Total	25	2	2	–	1	30

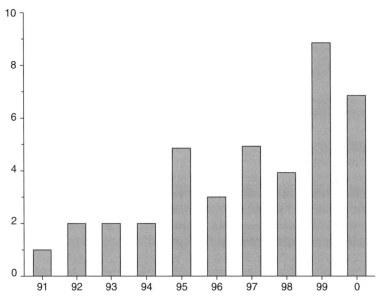

Figure 2. Number of prenatal investigations for HD in Denmark (1989 – 2000).

in at-risk couples, as many children of at-risk persons have been born during the period without a prenatal investigation. The number of prenatal investigations has been increasing during this period (*Figure 2*) but because of the small numbers it is difficult to state whether this increase is real.

All at-risk individuals in couples who applied for a prenatal test were Danish except for two Dutch males married and living in Denmark. Although the test is centralized, genetic counselling for HD is not. Most couples were given genetic counselling by a clinical geneticist, but in a few cases they were informed by an obstetrician.

Among the 30 couples there were more at-risk males than females, 18 versus 12, but the difference is not statistically significant. The mean age for the females at the time of the prenatal investigation was 26.7 years (range: 22–32) and for the males was 31.4 years (range: 27–51). Twenty of the 30 couples chose the direct test. In six cases the at-risk individual had been tested before the pregnancy, in nine the individual was tested during the pregancy, and five at-risk persons refused to be tested themselves. In two of the latter cases the prenatal test was positive, indirectly revealing that the at-risk parent also had the HD gene.

Prenatal testing was performed in 1 pregnancy in 25 couples. Repeated tests were performed in five couples with two, three and five consecutive pregnancies (*Table 5*). In one of these couples in which the woman was at risk, exclusion tests were performed in two consecutive pregnancies, whereas a direct test was performed in the other four cases of at-risk men, who had been previously tested positive.

An exclusion test was performed in 12 cases and in all a lowered risk for the fetus was encountered. This is not significantly different from the expected nine

Table 6. Results of prenatal investigations performed for Huntington's diseases in Denmark (1991–2000)

Risk	Exclusion test		Direct test		Total		Grand total
	Low	High	Low	High	Low	High	
Females	6	–	6	1	12	1	13
Males	6	–	10	11	16	11	27
Total	12	–	16	12	28	12	40

cases of low risk and three cases of high risk. Among the 28 fetuses that were tested directly, an increased risk was found in 12 and a lowered risk in 16 (*Table 6*).

All the pregnancies with a high risk for the fetus were terminated. This was the case for one of the couples who had three prenatal tests and for one with two prenatal tests. Both couples were then offered a preimplantation diagnostic genetic (PDG) test. Among the cases with a low risk for the fetus, one was aborted spontaneously, and in two other cases the pregnancies were terminated. In one case because a chromosome analysis revealed XXY, and in the other because a severe heart defect was found by ultrasound scanning of the fetus.

4.3 Prenatal testing for Huntington's disease in Denmark: discussion

As in other studies, we found that only a small percentage of at-risk persons makes use of prenatal investigation for HD. From our register we know that many children have been born to at-risk couples in whom prenatal investigation has not been performed. One reason for this may be that the at-risk persons do not know about that possibility. But even if at-risk individuals do know about prenatal investigations many prefer not to have it done. A most likely explanation may be that most people do not want to know about their gene status and are not aware of the exclusion test. Another explanation is that some of the couples are against abortion and may choose other options to prevent the birth of children with the HD gene. For instance, we know two couples who had an artificial insemination.

Nevertheless, the number of prenatal tests has shown an increasing trend during the 10 years that this procedure has been offered. The majority of the applicants for a prenatal test had not undergone a predictive test and so did not know their gene status. Ten of them chose the exclusion test, whereas others refused an exclusion test because of the 50% risk of the termination of a pregnancy with a fetus that does not have the HD gene. A third group of couples requested a predictive test before the prenatal investigation. They mentioned that they had earlier decided for a test but postponed it, but at that time felt that they should be tested before the fetus. Finally, a few at-risk couples insisted on having a prenatal test without a predictive test even though a positive result of the prenatal test would disclose that the at-risk parent is a gene carrier. Each single case is extremely difficult and complex regarding genetic counselling.

In our series, more couples with at-risk males applied for prenatal investigation than couples with at-risk females. This is in contrast to predictive testing where more women than men are usually tested. It is also striking that in four of the five couples that had consecutive prenatal tests, the man was the at-risk person. However, the numbers are small, so definite conclusions may not be drawn.

5. Prenatal testing for other late-onset neurogenetic disorders in Greece, Denmark, Germany, Austria and Switzerland

In all five countries, HD was the first late-onset neurogenetic disorder for which a prenatal test was performed, starting as early as 1991 in Greece and Denmark. Subsequently, molecular prenatal testing has become available in Greece for a number of other neurogenetic disorders, such as myotonic dystrophy (since 1994), Charcot-Marie-Tooth type I (since 1995) and spino-bulbar muscular atrophy (since 1993), all tested at the same unique Centre of Neurogenetics of the University of Athens (Yapijakis *et al.*, 1999; Yapijakis, unpublished data). The last disorder, known also as Kennedy syndrome, was tested in that centre for the first time universally (Yapijakis *et al.*, 1996).

In Denmark, a prenatal test for dentato-rubro-pallido-luysian atrophy in 1999 and one for Gerstmann-Straussler syndrome in 2001 have been performed, both probably for the first time in a Caucasian population (Sørensen, unpublished data). In the remaining three countries, there were no requests for prenatal diagnostic testing for other late-onset neurogenetic disorders.

References

Angastiniotis, M., Kyriakidou, S. and Hadjiminas M. (1988) The Cyprus thalassemia control program. *Birth Defects Orig. Artic. Ser.* **23(5B):** 417–432.

Conneally, P.M. (1984) Huntington disease: genetics and epidemiology. *Am. J. Hum. Genet.* **36:** 506–526.

Farrer, L., Myers, R., Cupples, L. and Conneally, P. (1988) Considerations in using linkage analysis as a presymptomatic test for Huntington disease. *J. Med. Genet.* **25:** 577–588.

Gusella, J.F., Wexler, N.S., Conneally, P.M., *et al* (1983) A polymorphic DNA marker genetically linked to Huntington's disease. *Nature* **306:** 234–238.

Harper, P.S., Lim, C. and Craufurd, D. (2000) Ten years of presymptomatic testing for Huntington's disease: the experience of the UK Huntington's Disease Prediction Consortium. *J. Med. Genet.* **37:** 567–571.

Harper, P.S., Morris, M. and Tyler, A. (1990) Genetic testing for Huntington's disease. *Br. Med. J.* **300:** 1089–1090.

Hayden, M., Kastelein, J., Wilson, R., Hilbert, C., Hewitt, J., Langlois, S., Fox, S. and Bloch, M. (1987) First trimester prenatal diagnosis for Huntington's disease with DNA probes. *Lancet* **1(8545):** 1284–1285.

Huntington's Disease Collaborative Research Group (1993) A novel gene containing a trinucleotide repeat that is expanded and unstable on Huntington's disease chromosomes. *Cell* **72:** 971–983.

International Huntington Association and World Federation of Neurology Research Group on Huntington's Chorea (1990) Ethical issues policy statement on Huntington's disease molecular genetics predictive test. *J. Med. Genet.* **27:** 334–338.

International Huntington Association and World Federation of Neurology Research Group on Huntington's Chorea (1994a) Guidelines for the molecular genetics predictive test in Huntington's disease. *J. Med. Genet.* **31:** 555–559.

International Huntington Association and World Federation of Neurology Research Group on Huntington's Chorea (1994b) Guidelines for the molecular genetics predictive test in Huntington's disease. *Neurology* **44:** 1533–1536.

Kanavakis, E., Traeger-Synodinos J., Vrettou, C., Maragoudaki, E., Tzetis, M. and Kattamis C. (1997) Prenatal diagnosis of the thalassaemia syndromes by rapid DNA analytical methods. *Mol. Hum. Reprod.* **3:** 523–528.

Kollia, P., Karababa, P.H., Sinopoulou, K., Voskaridou, E., Boussiou, M., Papadakis, M. and Loukopoulos, D. (1992) Beta-thalassaemia mutations and the underlying beta gene cluster haplotypes in the Greek population. *Gene Geogr.* **6:** 59–70.

Kreuz, F.R. (1996) Attitudes of German persons at risk for Huntington's disease toward predictive and prenatal testing. *Genet Couns.* **7:** 303–311.

Laccone, F., Engel, U., Holinski-Feder, E., et al (1999) DNA analysis of Huntington's disease: five years of experience in Germany, Austria, and Switzerland. *Neurology* **53:** 801–806.

Loukopoulos, D., Hadji, A., Papadakis, M., et al (1990) Prenatal diagnosis of thalassemia and of the sickle cell syndromes in Greece. *Ann. N.Y. Acad. Sci.* **612:** 226–236.

Loukopoulos, D., Karababa, P., Antsaklis, A., et al (1985) Prenatal diagnosis of thalassemia and Hb S syndromes in Greece: an evaluation of 1500 cases. *Ann. N.Y. Acad. Sci.* **445:** 357–375.

Maat-Kievit, A., Vegter-van der Vlis, M., Zoeteweij, M., Losekoot, M., van Haeringen, A. and Roos, R. (2000) Paradox of a better test for Huntington's disease. *J. Neurol. Neurosurg. Psychiat.* **69:** 579–583.

Mavrou, A., Metaxotou C. and Trichopoulos D. (1998) Awareness and use of prenatal diagnosis among Greek women: a national survey. *Prenat. Diagn.* **18:** 349–355.

Metaxotou C., Mavrou, A. and Antsaklis, A. (1997) Prenatal diagnosis services in Greece. *Eur. J. Hum. Genet.* **5(Suppl. 1):** 39–41.

Norremolle, A., Riess, O., Epplen, J.T., Fenger, K., Hashlt, L. and Sorensen, S.A. (1993) Trinucleotide repeat elongation in the Huntingtin gene in Huntington disease patients from 71 Danish families. *Hum. Molec. Genet.* **2:** 1475–1476.

Quarrell, O., Tyler, A., Upadhyaya, M., Meredith, A., Youngman, S. and Harper, P. (1987) Exclusion testing for Huntington's disease in pregnancy with a closely linked DNA marker. *Lancet* **1(8545):** 1281–1283.

Tzetis, M., Kanavakis, E., Antoniadi, T., Doudounakis, S., Adam, G. and Kattamis, C. (1997) Characterization of more than 85% of cystic fibrosis alleles in the Greek population, including five novel mutations. *Hum. Genet.* **99:** 121–125.

World Federation of Neurology Research Group on Huntington's Chorea (1993) Presymptomatic testing for Huntington's disease: a worldwide survey. *J. Med. Genet.* **30:** 1020–1022.

Yapijakis, C., Chronopoulou P., Prapas N., Vassilopoulos, D. and Papageorgiou, C. (1999) Prenatal diagnosis of myotonic dystrophy by fetal DNA testing. *Neurologia* **8:** 57–61.

Yapijakis, C., Kapaki, E., Boussiou, M., Vassilopoulos, D. and Papageorgiou, C. (1996) Prenatal diagnosis of X-linked spinal and bulbar muscular atrophy in a Greek family. *Prenat. Diagn.* **16:** 262–265.

Yapijakis, C., Loukopoulos, D., Metaxotou, C., Antsaklis, A. and Papageorgiou, C. (1993) Prenatal diagnosis of Huntington's chorea by fetal DNA testing. *Iatriki* **64:** 187–190.

Yapijakis, C., Vassilopoulos, D. and Papageorgiou, C. (1998) Predictive DNA testing for Huntington's disease: Attitudes of geneticists, neurologists and other spesialists. In: *Genetic Counseling in the Dawn of the 21st Century* (eds C. Bartsokas and P. Beighton). Zeta Publications, Athens, pp. 44–52.

Yapijakis, C., Vassilopoulos, D., Papageorgiou, C. and Loukopoulos, D. (1991) Presymptomatic diagnosis of Huntington's chorea in Greece. *Clin. Genet.* **40:** 91.

Yapijakis, C., Vassilopoulos, D., Tzagournissakis, M., Maris, T., Fesdjian, C., Papageorgiou, C. and Plaitakis, A. (1995) Linkage disequilibrium between the expanded

(CAG)n repeat and an allele of the adjacent (CCG)n repeat in Huntington's disease patients of Greek origin. *Eur. J. Hum. Genet.* **3**: 228–234.

Zuhlke, C., Riess, O., Schroder, K., Siedlaczck, I., Epplen, J.T., Engel, W. and Thies, U. (1993) Expansion of the (CAG)n repeat causing Huntington's disease in 352 patients of German origin. *Hum. Molec. Genet.* **2**: 1467–1469.

6

Legal aspects of prenatal testing for late-onset neurological diseases

Herman Nys, Carlos M. Romeo Casabona and
Christophe Desmet

1. Introduction

This chapter deals mainly with those legal aspects of prenatal testing that are most relevant for prenatal testing for late-onset neurogenetic diseases (in particular Huntington's disease). As a consequence of this focus it is obvious that not all the legal problems of prenatal testing or of genetic testing in general are dealt with.

In the following section, the legal protection of the unborn child and the termination of pregnancy are discussed. The subsequent section deals with the rights of the parents and the rights of the child (to be born). In the first subsection analysis is made of the parents' right to know by way of access to prenatal testing. The second subsection deals with the possible conflict between the right to know and the right not to know. In the final subsection we comment on the liability of the geneticist for wrongful birth and wrongful life, with particular attention to the recent legal developments in France.

2. Legal protection of the unborn child and termination of pregnancy

Although termination of pregnancy (TOP) is not a specific legal problem in prenatal testing for a late-onset disease, it is precisely in this particular case that the question arises whether TOP is lawful because the fetus will, if born alive,

Prenatal Testing for Late-Onset Neurogenetic Diseases, edited by G. Evers-Kiebooms, M. W. Zoeteweij and P. S. Harper

lead a 'normal' life for many years. In this chapter we first analyse the legal protection of the unborn child in international documents and the corresponding jurisprudence, and subsequently analyse the national legislation and jurisprudence regarding TOP in the case of a late-onset neurogenetic disease.

2.1 Legal protection of the unborn child in international law and its limits

The fundamental right to life is guaranteed in several international conventions, notably article 2 of the European Convention on Human Rights (ECHR) and article 6 of the International Convention on Civil and Political Rights. The right to life is considered a basic right, though not an absolute one, because article 2 ECHR tolerates infringement of this right in well-defined situations.

Moreover, the conventions do not explicitly define *from what moment* (conception?, implantation?, birth?) or *to what extent* the right to life is guaranteed. Article 2 ECHR, for instance, only stipulates that:

1. Everyone's right to life shall be protected by law. No one shall be deprived of his life intentionally save in the execution of a sentence of a court following his conviction of a crime for which this penalty is provided by law.
2. Deprivation of life shall not be regarded as inflicted in contravention of this article when it results from the use of force which is no more than absolutely necessary:
   a. in defence of any person from unlawful violence;
   b. in order to effect a lawful arrest or to prevent the escape of a person lawfully detained;
   c. in action lawfully taken for the purpose of quelling a riot or insurrection.

The European Commission for Human Rights has always avoided the question whether the unborn child is protected under article 2 ECHR, but the Commission was very explicit in excluding article 2 ECHR from granting the unborn child an absolute right to life under all circumstances, based on the fact that the mother also is entitled to the right to life. In a case in 1992 the Commission further stated that it would not exclude the possibility that under certain circumstances the article could be applicable to a fetus. The explicit position of the European Commission *against* granting the unborn child an *absolute* right to life has substantial legal importance. The rights of the unborn child are limited by the personality rights of the mother, namely, the right of the pregnant woman to have her physical integrity and her privacy respected (article 8 ECHR). This might be seen as an application of the principle of proportionality that runs as a constant theme throughout the entire Convention and its additional Protocols. Otherwise the compatibility between the different Member States' abortion legislation and the Convention could come under discussion, to the extent that it is not clear whether unborn life falls under the protection of article 2 ECHR. (In the supposition that article 2 ECHR would not concern the unborn child, the abortion legislation is of course juridicially allowed. Moreover, one could consider it as a desirable – albeit limited – extension of the right to life of the unborn child.) As already mentioned, not a single word about termination of pregnancy is mentioned in the enumerated exceptions to the right to life. From such a point of view abortion legislation can be seen as the legal clarification of the conditions under which the principle of proportionality is complied with, a principle whose concrete implementation falls under the 'margin of appreciation' of the Member States, within the context of the conflicting rights of mother and fetus.

2.2 Legal admissibility of termination of pregnancy in the case of a late-onset disease

Prenatal diagnosis may alleviate a couples' or a woman's anxiety about giving birth to seriously ill or severely disabled children, and from that point of view it provides an answer to a real social demand. It can also be a vital aid in monitoring pregnancies for therapeutic reasons with a view to safe deliveries. Nevertheless, most prenatal diagnosis is performed in order to prevent the birth of disabled children: with current medical knowledge, fetal treatment is seldom an option. In the case of most tests, abortion is an integral part of the whole procedure, and the revelation of illness or disability in the fetus confronts the couple or the woman with the choice of whether to continue or to terminate the pregnancy. This brings us to one of the major legal issues involving prenatal diagnosis: under what conditions is TOP allowed?

A distinction is made according to the moment at which the TOP is performed. So-called late TOP during the second trimester of the pregnancy, in most countries, after the 12th week of gestation, is far more strictly regulated than TOP during the first trimester. For this reason we concentrate upon the normative framework concerning *late* TOP. (It must be noted that the Begian law on TOP (just like other abortion laws) speaks of the 12th week from conception. It is not quite clear whether this moment also counts as the starting point for the calculation of the so-called 'week of gestation', a notion that often comes up in the literature. In general, a pregnancy of 12 weeks means that 12 weeks have passed since the last menstruation, whereas the conception only takes place 14 days later. The difference between the two criteria can be up to 2 weeks, which can be particularly relevant from a juridicial point of view.)

Belgium. In Belgium, TOP is regulated in the articles 350 (2) and following of the Criminal Code, as enacted by the law of 3 April 1990. Article 350 (2) 4° contains additional stipulations to the general conditions concerning a TOP during the first trimester (situation of distress, firm will and explicit request of the woman, TOP performed by a physician, in an institute for health care with an information service, counselling and a waiting period of 6 days), which have to be fulfilled in order for a TOP after the 12th week of gestation not to be punishable. First, the pregnancy must be such that its continuation would seriously endanger the woman's health or that it is *indisputable* that the expected child will certainly suffer from a particularly serious condition, considered as incurable at the time of the diagnosis. Besides that, the collaboration of a second physician, whose advice has to be added to the medical record, is obligatory. In the following section, we concentrate on the legal questions arising from the first (additional) condition, and more precisely on the question whether the situation of a fetus carrying the gene for a late-onset disease, such as Huntington's disease (HD), can be considered as a situation that would legitimate a termination of pregnancy.

It is beyond all doubt that HD is a *'particularly serious condition'*, which is also incurable at present. The problem is the time-frame: at which moment, at the moment of birth, or at an indefinite moment somewhere in the future, does the child need to suffer from the illness in order to fulfil the first condition? From the first point of view (the illness has to exist at the moment of birth) no legal TOP after the 12th week is possible for HD, precisely because of the late-onset character of the disease. In other words, the child does not *suffer* from the disease at the moment of birth, and will have many years of asymptomatic life. However, one can criticize this restrictive vision, because nowhere does the law *explicitly* exclude that it is sufficient that the child will with certainty suffer from the disease, albeit at an unknown moment in the future, for the disease to be considered incurable at the moment of diagnosis. An alternative solution can be found in directly appealing to the *'danger for the health of the woman'*, in which case it is not her physical but her mental health that would be endangered, because her pregnancy could be particularly aggravating because of her knowledge that the fetus is carrying the Huntington mutation.

Finally, the question remains up until what moment after the 12th week of gestation TOP should be allowed (whether for HD or not). In Belgian law, there is no reference whatsoever to a period during which TOP is or is not allowed. During parliamentary debates, however, a restrictive definition of the notion 'TOP' was given: the viability of the fetus constitutes the ultimate limit. TOP is therefore limited to the non-viable fetus.

France (article L.2212–1–article L.2223–2 Code de la santé publique).   Since the Law of 4 July 2001, TOP in France is considered as 'late' from the 12th week of pregnancy. After this point, TOP is only allowed, regardless of the general conditions for a TOP during the first trimester, when the continuation of the pregnancy may seriously endanger the (physical and/or mental) health of the woman, or when it is *highly probable* that the child to be born will be affected by a particular serious incurable disorder recognized as such at the time of diagnosis. Moreover, the confirmation of one of these indications by two physicians is obligatory. Although French law on TOP closely resembles Belgian law, an important difference between them is that in France *a high probability* with regard to the seriousness of the disorder and its incurable character is sufficient, whereas the Belgian law requires that *both the seriousness and the incurable character of the illness are established*. Concerning the intervention of the second physician, French law, in its turn, is more stringent than Belgian law because it requires the confirmation of the indication by two physicians who are specialists in that field, whereas in Belgium the advice of a second physician, not necessarily a specialist, is sufficient.

Finally, it is remarkable that there is no final limit for a late TOP in France. The law allows TOP *'à toute époque'* (at any moment in time) regardless of the term of the pregnancy or the developmental stage of the unborn child.

Germany. In Germany TOP is dealt with in the Law of 27 July 1992, as amended by the Law of 21 August 1995, which classified the regulation of TOP under article 218–219b *Strafgesetzbuch*. TOP after the 12th week is allowed in Germany, in cases of so-called '*mütterlich medizinische Indikation*', without any restriction in time, and without any obligatory counselling. This '*maternal medical indication*' refers to a situation in which TOP is necessary to prevent a threat to the life of the pregnant woman or a threat of serious injury to her physical or mental health. The former law of 1992 also contained a stipulation explicitly speaking of an irremediable injury to the child to be born (the so-called embryo-pathological/fetopathological indication), to such a degree that one could not request that the mother would have to carry out her pregnancy. In 1995 this indication was abolished, and this raises the question of whether this indication is still in force under the new law. A realistic interpretation is that this indication has been encompassed by the *maternal medical indication*. This has important consequences. The application of maternal indication was limited to an actual danger to the life or health of the mother during pregnancy, and a severely handicapped fetus could not be considered as a danger in this sense. Indeed, the former fetopathological indication did not aim to offer protection to the mother for the physical damage caused *before* the birth of a handicapped child, but only protection to the costs and care *after* the birth of a handicapped child. Under the new law, the application of the maternal indication is much broader and also justifies an abortion when the continuation of the pregnancy has become unbearable because of a severe fetal handicap.

The Netherlands. The law of 1 May 1981, amended by the law of 28 January 1999, regulates TOP in The Netherlands. Unlike all the other laws on TOP, this law makes no distinction between so-called 'early' or 'late' TOP: in both cases the decision to terminate the pregnancy has to be taken with the necessary due care, and it will only be performed if the woman's situation of distress is firmly and invariably established. Counselling is obligatory and there is also a waiting period of 6 days provided in the law.

With regard to the final limit for a TOP, we refer to article 82(a) of the Criminal Code: '*With depriving another, or a child at the moment of birth or directly thereafter, of his life, is meant: the killing of a fetus which may reasonably be assumed to be capable of remaining alive outside the mother's body.*' Such an act does not constitute termination of pregnancy, but falls under the range of application of infanticide in article 287–291 of the Criminal Code. The Dutch legislator has *explicitly* equated the killing of a fetus, once it has reached the stage of viability, with infanticide.

United Kingdom. In the United Kingdom, the Abortion Act 1967, as amended by article 37 of the Human Fertilisation and Embryology act 1990, allows TOP as long as the pregnancy is terminated by a registered medical practitioner and as long as two registered medical practitioners are of the opinion, formed in good faith, that:

(a) the pregnancy has *not exceeded its 24th week*, and that the continuation of the pregnancy would involve a greater risk than if the pregnancy were terminated, of injury to the physical or mental health of the *pregnant woman or any existing children of her family*; or

(b) the TOP is necessary in order to prevent *grave permanent injury* to the physical or mental health of *the pregnant woman*; or

(c) the continuation of the pregnancy would involve greater *risk to the life of the pregnant woman* than if the pregnancy were terminated; or

(d) there is a substantial risk that *if the child were born* it would suffer from such physical or mental abnormalities as to be seriously handicapped.

Section d is concerned with the life of the 'child' if born. Consequently, the condition must exist after birth at some point. However, to require the condition, and its manifestation, to exist at the point of birth or immediately thereafter is too narrow a reading of the law. A reasonable interpretation would allow the doctor to project forward during the child's life, if born, and assess what its condition would be and whether it would suffer 'serious handicap'. Of course there must be 'physical or mental abnormality' during this time. This would not be broad enough to cover the case of a carrier of a defective gene, which did not manifest itself in the child, for example, a recessive condition such as *cystic fibrosis*. However, some conditions do not manifest themselves and so lead to 'serious handicap' until much later in the child's life, for example HD. Are these within the scope of section 1 (1) d? On one view they are not. The Act speaks of the 'child', if born, suffering from 'such physical or mental abnormalities as to be seriously handicapped'. HD does not usually manifest itself until a person is in his or her 40s. Only a broad construction of 'child' could encompass this situation. And, although it is difficult on the wording of section 1 (1) d to include conditions in adulthood, once it is accepted that the handicap need not manifest itself at birth, it would seem to undermine the purpose of the principle to restrict it narrowly to childhood (Grubb, 1998).

With regard to actual medical practice, Harper and Taylor (1991) state that 'although most TOP are meant for disorders causing serious handicap *in early life*, it seems unlikely that a request from a person carrying a pregnancy at risk for HD would be refused' (p. 354: note that this statement dates from the period wherein only DNA linkage was possible).

In cases b, c and d, TOP is possible after the 24th week, without any time limit. Neither counselling nor a waiting period is imposed by the Abortion Act 1967.

Sweden. The Swedish Law of 18 May 1995 amended the Abortion Law of 14 June 1974. According to this law we speak of a late TOP after the 18th week of pregnancy. After the 18th week of pregnancy, an abortion may only be performed if sanctioned by the National Board of Health and Welfare, irrespective of the stage the pregnancy has reached, provided that it is deemed that the pregnancy, by reason of a disease or physical defect of the woman, is likely to entail a serious risk to her life or health.

Denmark. TOP is allowed in Denmark after the 12th week in the following exceptional circumstances (see section 3 of the Law of 1973):

(a) when there are social reasons for the woman;

(b) when the pregnancy was caused by rape or incest;

(c) when the child is endangered because of hereditary problems or sickness during the embryonic stage;
(d) at any time, when there is serious risk to the woman's health or life.

[See the law on the termination of pregnancy of 13 June 1973, as promulgated by Order No. 633 of 15 September 1986 and as most recently amended by Law No. 389 of 14 June 1995, is further amended by: the insertion of a new subsection 3 in Sec. 3, which deals with termination after the 12th week of pregnancy, which states that, if the fetus is deemed to be viable, termination may be permitted only if the circumstances referred to in point 3 of subsection 1 ('when there is a danger that, on account of a hereditary condition or of an injury or disease during embryonic or foetal life, the child will be affected by a serious physical or mental disorder') are sufficiently important to justify it; and the insertion of a new subsection 4 in Sec. 8, which prescribes that counselling should be offered to the woman before and after the intervention (detailed rules are to be determined by the Minister of Justice). Law No. 430 of 31 May 2000 amending the Law on the termination of pregnancy (late induced abortions).]

Norway. In Norway a distinction is made between the first period of 12 weeks, the second period from the 12th to the 18th week, and a third period after the 18th week of pregnancy. After the 12th week and before the 18th week of pregnancy has elapsed, the pregnancy may be terminated with the permission of a Medical Board of two physicians, who can take quite a broad range of grounds into account. After the 18th week of pregnancy has elapsed, TOP can be performed only if there are particularly important grounds for doing so. If there is reason to believe that the fetus is viable, authorization for a TOP shall not be granted. In cases, however, where the pregnancy constitutes an impending risk to the woman's life or health, it may be terminated at any time.

Finland. A pregnancy may be terminated between 12 and 20 weeks of gestation with permission from the National Board of Medico-legal Affairs, if the woman has not attained the age of 17 at the time of conception or if there are other special grounds for doing so.

TOP is also allowed before the 24th week of gestation, with permission from the National Board of Medico-legal Affairs if tests show that the fetus is seriously ill, or has a serious physical deformity.

When the continuation of the pregnancy or the delivery of a child, because of the woman's illness, physical deformity or infirmity, would endanger her life or health, a pregnancy may be interrupted at any time, by any physician.

Spain. Spanish abortion law is very strict, even during the first 12 weeks of gestation: abortion during the first 12 weeks is only allowed when the pregnancy is the consequence of rape. After the 12th week, TOP can only be performed:

(a) to avert a serious risk to the physical or mental health of the pregnant woman (no time limit); or
(b) when it is presumed that the fetus if borne to term, would suffer from severe physical or mental defects (provided that the abortion is performed within the first 22 weeks of pregnancy).

Portugal. TOP is possible *at any time* if it is the only means of preventing the death or serious and irreversible damage to the physical or mental health of the mother.

Within 24 weeks, TOP can be performed if there is a serious malformation of the fetus or if the new-born will suffer a serious incurable disease.

If the pregnancy is the result of rape, the pregnancy can be terminated *before the 16th week* of gestation.

When there is a serious risk to the woman's physical or mental health, TOP is possible *within the first 12 weeks*.

Consent for TOP may not be given less than 3 days prior to the interruption of pregnancy.

In January 1998, the Portuguese parliament voted in favour of liberalizing the law on abortion so as to permit unrestricted access to abortion in pregnancies of up to 10 weeks. However, because of the importance and sensitivity of the matter, the political parties agreed to put it to a referendum. In the referendum on 28 June 1998, the people voted by a narrow majority against such a change in the law.

Greece. The Law of 28 June 1986 on voluntary termination of pregnancy allows TOP after the 12th week in the following cases:

(a) the fetus suffers from a serious abnormality that will result in a serious congenital defect (before 24th week); or
(b) there is an unavoidable risk to the life of the woman or to serious and permanent harm to her physical or mental health (no time limit); or
(c) in cases of rape, incest, or when the woman is a minor (19 weeks of gestation).

There is no waiting period imposed.

Italy. Here also a distinction is made between the first period of 12 weeks, and the period after the 12th week of gestation, but here the law speaks of days (90), not of weeks, so in fact the first period counts 12 weeks and 6 days. Late termination of pregnancy is allowed in following situations:

(a) when the pregnancy or childbirth entails a serious threat to the woman's life, except when the fetus is already viable;
(b) when serious abnormalities or malformations of the fetus constitute a serious threat to the physical/mental health of the woman;
(c) when the pregnancy is the result of rape.

Luxembourg. After a delay of 12 weeks, an interruption of pregnancy will only be possible if two qualified medical doctors ascertain in a written statement that there exists a serious risk to the health of the pregnant woman or the child-to-be.

2.3 Closing comments regarding the legal protection of the unborn child and termination of pregnancy

It is not easy to draw general conclusions from this survey of national legislation on late TOP. However, some striking features are the following. First, it is clear that with the possible exception of the law in the UK, national legislatures have not taken into account a late-onset disease as a distinct indication for a late TOP. This is not surprising given the fact that most of these laws already existed when prenatal testing for a late-onset disease became possible. Second, most laws provide for a fetal indication that allows a late TOP but, with the exception of the UK law, it is far from clear whether the legislature has implied that this indication also applies when the fetus is the carrier of mutation at the origin of a severe late-onset disease. Sometimes it is clear that the law requires that the disease already exists *in utero* or, at the latest, at the moment of birth (see for instance the Portuguese or the Italian law). In other laws the application to late-onset diseases is doubtful although not excluded explicitly (see for instance the Belgian and French laws). Third, in countries where there is certainty or serious doubt about whether the fetal indication is applicable, a late TOP after the prenatal diagnosis of a late-onset disease is only permitted when a broad interpretation of the maternal indication is taken. This means that the knowledge that one is pregnant with a fetus that carries a mutation at the origin of a late-onset disease is a severe danger for the mental health of the pregnant woman. Whether this interpretation corresponds with what the legislature had in mind at the moment the law was written is not at all certain.

3. The rights of the parents and the child

Do parents have a right to claim a genetic test? This question is a general one and does not concern prenatal diagnosis alone, but all kinds of (predictive) genetic diagnosis. The fundamental question here is whether the 'right to know' is a sufficient legal basis to claim the carrying out of (predictive) genetic diagnosis.

3.1 The right to know and access to prenatal testing

The 'right to know' is recognized in article 10.2. of the European Convention for the Protection of Human Rights and Dignity of the Human Being with Regard to the Application of Biology and Medicine (ECRMBio), which stipulates that '*everyone is entitled to know any information collected about his or her health.*' The Convention speaks of the right to know any information *collected* about his or her health, but does not deal with the question whether this right to know also includes one's right to request that information about his or her (future) health be generated. The 'mirror-image' of this right, i.e. the 'right not to know', is also guaranteed under the same article of the Convention. Gevers states that this 'right not to know' not only aims at the possibility of being spared, if one so desires, from already available information concerning his health status, but it also includes the right to determine by oneself whether that information *may* be generated (European Court of Justice, 1994). This argues that the right to know also includes the right to know information not yet generated. In other words, the right to know, in this view, constitutes a solid legal basis to obtain access to information about one's genetic constitution or one's (future) health status, and more specifically to claim the carrying out of a genetic test, without interference by the government or by others, especially the physician.

Before starting this analysis, another important problem has to be raised. It concerns the question whether a pregnant woman needs the father's consent for a genetic test on her fetus *in utero*, because one of the father's parents has HD, or whether this test can lawfully be done without his consent. The major problem in such a case is that a positive test on the fetus also indicates that the father has the mutation and will develop the disease later in life. This is knowledge that many people do not want to have (Skene, 2001).

The question then arises whether clinicians confronted with a pregnant woman wanting to have her fetus tested, in the absence of the father's involvement in this procedure, should allow the test to be carried out. It is remarkable that clinical practice in Australia is more restrictive than what Australian law in this area requires. Many clinicians only allow the test if the father consents. This point of view is inspired by the concern to avoid serious problems in the family later on, but also by the concern that the father should not have to receive such devastating news from the mother, explicitly or implicitly, without adequate medical and psychological counselling and support at that moment. The IHA-WFN Guidelines mentioned above deal with these concerns, particularly in the comments on point 7.1 : 'It is highly desirable that both parents agree to an antenatal test. If there is a conflict, every effort should be made by the counsellors and the couple to reach an agreement. Exceptional circumstances (e.g. rape or incest) may justify deviating from this recommendation.'

However, from a legal point of view, there are no specific principles that require the father's active participation in this field, as only the mother is a patient in this case, and the duty to take reasonable care, which includes informed consent, is only owed to the patient, not to other parties. But the duty of informed consent may include advice regarding other family members (although there's no separate duty to family members) as the duty of informed consent is a duty to give a patient all relevant information in order to make an autonomous decision whether to proceed with a medical act. When being counselled about the potential implications of a positive test result, the mother, therefore, should also be informed about the possible effect on the father.

The right to know and interference by the government.   Roscam Abbing and Gevers (1996) argue that the right to know *as such* does not constitute a sufficient legal basis for claiming genetic testing, but it might do so in combination with other rights, for instance the social right to health care (article 3 ECHRBio). Insofar as predictive genetic diagnosis serves the purposes of health, it falls under the scope of the right to health care. However, when the (predictive) genetic diagnosis serves interests other than the examined person's (future) health or the interests of others, requests for genetic testing will not have a strong enough basis to require the government and the community to comply with these claims. This right to health care involves the government's commitment to undertake all necessary efforts for the protection and the promotion of public health, and that there be a minimum of genetic services available and accessible for everyone without discrimination or financial constraints (European Group on Ethics in Science and New Technologies, 1996; World Health Organization, 1997). This includes the development of incentives to ensure that appropriate genetic diagnostic technologies are developed and that the use of the above-mentioned diagnostic technologies is allowed (Andrews, 1990).

Specific to those genetic diagnostic procedures related to reproduction decision-making (prenatal, preconceptional and preimplantation diagnosis), a couple's right to procreative freedom (derived from article 8 and 12 ECHR) should also be taken into account, besides their right to know. Does a couple's right to reproduce or to avoid reproduction give them a right of access to genetic testing? Of course, this right does not include a claim for a child, but implies that no one may obstruct them in their decision-making process. The question remains, however, whether the right to procreative liberty which forbids interference by others, especially the government, in one's reproductive decision-making process, also obliges the government to provide active support, by way of access to (predictive) genetic diagnosis, in this decision-making process (Royal College of Physicians, 1991). Some authors argue that, even without a medical indication or purpose, (predictive) genetic diagnosis cannot simply be forbidden (Guldix, 1993–94), and if there are genetic services available, they should be accessible to anyone, without discrimination.

The right to know and interference by the physician.   With reference to the World Health Organization's definition of 'health', one could argue that even without a medical indication, a physician could not refuse a request to undergo a medical intervention, because there might always be some psychological or social indication for the applicant. However, when we look at the origin of this broad interpretation of the notion 'health', the 19th century public health movement, it turns out that this was meant as an incentive *for national governments* to promote the health and the welfare of their citizens. Applying this broad philosophical, rather than legal, definition to the particular patient–physician relation would not only be historically inaccurate, it would also lead towards over-medicalization, stimulating patients to claim any 'medical' intervention whatsoever from a physician.

It is our belief that, in the particular patient–physician relation, physicians must have and indeed do have some kind of counterweight at their disposal by which they can decide themselves whether to comply with a request for an intervention, for instance a request for (predictive) genetic diagnosis. A patient's right to know, though embedded in the right to respect private life and hence broadly interpretable, forms as such no solid and self-sufficient legal basis for claims to knowledge about one's medical condition. It belongs in the first place to the physician's professional autonomy to determine under which circumstances a medical intervention is necessary or useful for the promotion of one's health. That counterweight can be found in the physician's so-called *diagnostic and therapeutic liberty or professional autonomy*. Once a legal relationship between a patient and a physician has originated, the patient has a right to careful medical treatment. However, the physician is free to choose all means he or she deems necessary to make a diagnosis or to carry out a treatment. It is the physician who decides whether some diagnostic test is medically indicated. The physician has to be considered as the 'medical gatekeeper', deciding under what conditions illness, as a reason for accessing healthcare services, justifies a medical intervention.

That professional autonomy, however, is not absolute: a physician might incur liability, civil, criminal or disciplinary, when he or she deviates from the so-called professional medical standard of due care. To make this abstract 'professional medical standard of due care' concrete, judges often rely on practice that is customary among physicians. Thus the generally approved practice of the profession plays an important role in the judge's decision-making process, but not a decisive one. This is called the *normative aspect* of the standard of due care: a physician does not apply the due care which is *customary* in the medical profession, but the due care which can be *expected* of a physician of the same skill, placed in the same circumstances. Nevertheless, judges often refer to medical protocols, recommendations, guidelines, standards and so on that serve as an initial guideline for their judgement.

More specifically, when a physician is confronted with a request for prenatal testing, he or she will have to decide whether to comply with it, and this decision must be based on what a standard physician with the same competence, placed in the same circumstances, would do. He or she can therefore rely on the common practice as described in protocols, guidelines, advices, etc., such as the International Huntington's Association and World Federation of Neurology Guidelines (1994).

In numerous other international professional codes of conduct we encounter 'medical indication' as a requirement for prenatal genetic testing, in view of reducing the risk of eugenics (see also Chapter IV of the ECHRBio). In this context it is worth examining point 2.7 of the *Opinion on Ethical Aspects of Prenatal Diagnosis* of 20 February 1996 of the *European Group on Ethics in Science and New Technologies*, where we find a clear demand for a specific medical indication. Another example can be found in the Recommendation R(90)13 of the Committee of Ministers of the Council of Europe from 21 June 1990, which recommends the use of prenatal diagnosis and prenatal screening only for medical purposes. In the *Proposed International Guidelines on Ethical Issues in Medical Genetics and Genetic Services* (1997) of the World Heath Organization, it is clearly stated that the use of prenatal diagnosis for paternity testing or for gender selection, apart from sex-linked disorders, is unacceptable, and that prenatal diagnosis solely to alleviate maternal anxiety, *in the absence of medical indications*, should have lower priority in the allocation of resources than prenatal diagnosis with medical indications.

The professional standard of care implies that prenatal diagnosis will essentially be reserved exclusively for '*medical indications*', so that it cannot be used to obtain information about medically non-relevant characteristics. When there is *no indication at all* (such as previous familial history, age of the mother, deformity visualized through ultrasound scanning) physicians usually will not perform the prenatal diagnosis on the request of the parents alone, as in such cases the right-not-to-know and the future child's right to privacy are also at stake. But even when there is a medical indication, the same conflict of rights between parents and the future child will arise. In practice, there are physicians who try to deal with this problem by allowing the prenatal diagnosis only on the condition that the woman will undergo a TOP if the testing shows an unfavourable result. In this case the question arises, not whether this is legally *admissible*, but whether this is legally *possible*. And for more than one reason, the answer to this question has to be a negative one.

First of all, such a request will never be enforceable if the woman decided not to have a TOP. The physician who deliberately performs a TOP on a woman against her will commits a criminal offence. Another reason to deny the possibility of this condition is that this would constitute discrimination against women who have a different motive for undergoing a prenatal diagnosis than the termination of the pregnancy in the case of a disorder, for instance, because they want to be (psychologically) prepared for the birth of a handicapped child. But it also constitutes discrimination against the future child for whom the result of the testing is not (sufficiently) unfavourable to let the condition become 'operative'. In this case the dilemma still remains. Subsequently, the question arises, what is to be considered as an *'unfavourable result'*, which triggers the condition, and who determines the content of this notion?

Nevertheless, although this requirement of TOP is unacceptable in general, we think that in the context of HD it exhibits a certain usefulness. Notwithstanding the fact that refusing the test to the parents might be an infringement of their right to know and their right to health care, precisely because there is a medical indication, the refusal seems to be justified because of the fact that HD is a late-onset disease, so that the parents have no legitimate interest in the information: on the one hand, they are not willing to undergo a TOP; on the other hand, in case of HD there is (as yet) no possibility to provide early medication aimed at preventing or postponing the symptoms. In such a case the interest of the parents would seem to have less weight than the interest of the child to choose, once it is competent, whether it wants the information concerning its health situation. It would be different in the case of a handicap that is present at birth: in such a case, the parents could invoke other reasons in support of their right to know.

3.2 The right to know versus the right not to know

It is clear that there needs to be a discussion about the relevance of both the right to be informed (especially when it requires information from a third party) and the right to refuse any kind of information (Fedder, 2000; Porn, 1997), particularly when the subjects of both rights are members of the same family, in which there is a deleterious gene responsible for a serious disease, as in the case of HD.

The right to be informed (right to know). The right to know, or the right to receive information, is nowadays recognized as one of the most important rights of the patient, whether it is related to consent to medical treatment. As already mentioned, article 10.2 ECHRBio explicitly recognizes this right.

Closely connected with the right to receive information about one's health is the right to keep such information away from third parties. Article 10.1 of the

ECHRBio recognizes the right to respect for one's private life in relation to information about one's health. The European Union's Directive on the subject (European Parliament and Council, 2000) must also be borne in mind (article 8). However, the special nature of individual genetic data requires special protection and one has to ask whether already existing instruments satisfy this need. There is no doubt that medical and nursing staff have a duty of confidentiality concerning the outcomes of genetic tests performed and other information collected by them (Nielsen, 1996; Taupitz, 1996). As has rightly been said, an important measure for protecting confidentiality lies in affording greater protection to medical records in general and in reducing the relevance of those records to coverage for health care (Yesley, 1997). Another way of thinking, which is finding increasing support, is that each person is also entitled to decide to whom, when and to what extent such information can be disclosed. Thus, the passing on of information obtained by means of genetic testing should be prohibited unless consent is given by the person to which the data belong or by the legal representative in the case of minors or legally incapacitated persons.

The right to ignorance (right not to know). In connection with the right to information, or right to know, mention is often made of the emergence of the opposing right, that is, the 'right not to know' (Cavoukian, 1995; Rodota, 1990; Taupitz, 1998). This is a right that has arisen essentially in the field of genetic information, although also with similar controversy in other health areas (De Sola, 1994; Rodota, 1990; Romeo Casabona, 1994; Roscam Abbing, 1995). This right has been expressly recognized by article 10.2 of the ECHRBio: everyone has the right not to be informed.

This right not to know means that by not undergoing genetic testing the subject avoids knowing whether he or she is carrying a mutation that causes a genetic condition or whether he or she is going to suffer from a genetic condition in the future. This attitude might be viewed as selfish and irresponsible (see, for arguments against this right, which should be contrary to the ethics of responsibility, in a sense close to Hans Jonas's Theory of Responsibility – Das Prinzip Verantwortung: Hottois, 1999. See also other arguments against it, with comments by Chadwick, 1997) if it serves to block scientific progress or prevent family members or future offspring from being conscious of the condition. It could therefore be countered by coercive measures backed by law. However, it should be pointed out that anyone who tries to invoke the so-called 'right not to know' (a right of which he or she may probably be unaware) starts from the position that he or she 'already knows'. The explicit wish not to undergo testing implies that the individual already knows that he or she belongs to a genetic disease risk group or at least is aware of a similar previous history in members of the family; he or she may even know that science does not have adequate means to prevent, treat, diminish or mitigate the genetic disease. In this context the person may choose not to receive further information (i.e. as to whether he or she is carrying a deleterious gene or is going to suffer a disease), particularly if the disease is highly serious, in order to avoid this knowledge from altering his or her personal development and social advancement from that moment onwards. One prefers not to be aware of something which science can do nothing to alleviate.

Consequently, the right to protection of a private life free from external intrusion re-emerges today as the guarantee of a decision taken individually, based on the understanding that the right not to know is merely a manifestation of the right to privacy and of the respect for one's private life (Martinez-Bullé Goyri, 1995).

Conflicting situations: the right not to know versus the right to know.   Genetic data must also be protected *vis-à-vis* other persons even in the case of a biological relative who seeks information concerning the possible presence in him or her of a pathological gene similar to that discovered in the data subject, and inherited from the parents (The Danish Council of Ethics, 1993), or when the physician considers it necessary for family members to know the information because they might also be affected by the results of the genetic test. The European Commission's Group of Advisers on the Ethical Implications of Biotechnology (1996) insists on the need for maintaining confidentiality in these cases as well.

One frequently observes, however, that the subject consents to the disclosure of information to members of the family or may even provide the information himself (De Sola, 1994). Moreover, in genetic counselling the subject should recognize the importance, for others (family), of partially relieving the physician of his professional duty of secrecy, or of giving the information directly himself (Annas *et al.*, 1995).

It is worth dwelling for a moment on some of the conflict situations that could arise as a result of reproduction related diagnosis. In many cases, physicians find themselves in an awkward position when diagnosis confirms the existence, in the person(s) seeking the counselling, of pathological genes that might transmit hereditary disorders to offspring. Should physicians disclose the risk personally to family members or should they trust that the persons seeking the counselling will do so, and thus enable the family members to seek appropriate advice or preventive measures? Bear in mind that if the family members in question are children, they will be most at risk, given that the deleterious gene may not yet have manifested itself and hence the disease may be in the presymptomatic stage or the person's predisposition may not yet be obvious. Knowledge of such a situation would be crucial in order to enable them to be treated adequately, though unfortunately there is in some cases no effective treatment, as is the case for HD.

Possible solutions and some comments.   Once the relevance and the legal protection of the aforementioned rights have been settled, restrictions on all of them are possible in some circumstances. For the purposes of our considerations here, the relevant provisions of the ECHRBio for establishing possible restrictions are the following: 'no restrictions shall be placed on the exercise of the rights and protective provisions contained in this Convention other than such as are prescribed by law and are necessary in a democratic society in the interest of public safety, for the prevention of crime, for the protection of public health or for the protection of the rights and freedoms of others' (article 26). The problem will be to specify when the rights and freedoms of others should prevail.

In fact, it is possible to consider the interests of third parties, when their life or health can be seriously affected without a specific legal regulation, by calling on the so-called 'collision of duties' (Roscam Abbing, 1995). See also Malem Seña (1995) (as a principles collision). The Nuffield Council on Bioethics (1993) also admits some exceptions to the duty of confidentiality or, alternatively, on 'the state of necessity'.

In the former case (collision of duties), a person, in this case a physician, is in a situation where two legal duties are in conflict: the obligation of confidentiality towards his own patient, and the obligation to protect the life or health of another (e.g., a relative of the patient). The legal result is that, no matter what course of action is adopted, he will always contravene one of the two obligations, because they are incompatible with each other, and the most important obligation in the concrete case should be fulfilled. In the latter case (state of necessity), there is no conflict between two obligations, but an obligation is contravened in order to avoid a grave danger to another person towards whom there is no legal obligation (e.g. the obligation of confidentiality towards the patient is contravened by the physician faced with a predictable danger for a family member with whom there is no professional relation at all).

The techniques used to solve these sorts of conflicts are well known by the majority of jurisdictions: to solve the problem correctly, all the interests present in the problem have to be considered. The weighing of interests has to be done with objective criteria (Cerezo Mir, 1998). In order to apply the first alternative, i.e. collision of duties, it is necessary that the existence of an obligation of information towards the third person be previously determined (even if this is a relative of the person that has the right to confidentiality). Nevertheless, it is believed that the existence of such an obligation will only occur in very exceptional cases (Annas et al., 1995). Regarding the second alternative, the state of necessity, it will be very important to show that the knowledge of a person's genetic data will be decisive to be able to diagnose prematurely another illness and to immediately initiate a more or less effective treatment to prevent, cure or alleviate a serious illness or to delay its onset. In the case of illnesses for which at present there is no effective treatment or ways of avoiding or delaying its onset, it will be difficult to show the prevailing interest of the right to be informed. This is the case with HD. In that case, it should be proved that the premature detection of a person as presymptomatic carrier could be of great importance, at least in delaying its appearance or its most serious symptoms.

Data protection and professional secrecy requirements extend to each individual's genetic information, and it is up to the individual to decide how, to whom and to what extent such information should be disclosed. Thus, the passing on to others of information obtained via genome analysis is prohibited unless consent is given by the person concerned or by his legal representatives. Where a conflict of interest arises because a member of the affected person's family requests information in order to know whether a pathological gene similar to the one discovered in the patient and inherited from the parents might be also present in him, this rule may admit exceptions. But we have seen that this is only valid in a few cases (Bompiani, 2001).

Finally, these problems are the evidence that genetic information is in need of a better and more accurate regulation and protection, taking into account all the interests involved.

3.3 Liability of the geneticist for wrongful birth and wrongful life

The possibility of genetic diagnosis also raises questions concerning civil liability. In the case of prenatal (and also preimplantation or preconceptional) diagnosis, negligent medical action may often lead towards a very particular situation, in which the birth of a child with a handicap is qualified as damage. In such cases, the parents may sue the physician because of the '*unlawful birth*' of their handicapped child. Such a claim is being called the '*Wrongful Birth*' claim. This has come over from certain common-law countries into Western European countries. The success of such actions depends on the presence of the standard elements of a tort claim, more precisely that there is a legal *duty of care* owed to the plaintiffs, that there was a *breach* of that duty by conduct failing to reach the professional standard of care and skill and that they suffered a legally recognized *injury, caused by the breach* of the duty of care. But first we must distinguish a variety of related legal claims, which often tend to be confused, in the field of actions for damages by children and parents arising from occurrences before birth.

We can speak of *a wrongful conception or a wrongful pregnancy claim* when a parent brings a claim following negligence that has led to the birth of an unwanted *healthy* child. This claim may arise typically in two situations, namely where the negligence relates to contraceptive advice or treatment (failed sterilization) or where the negligence involves a failed abortion carried out to prevent the birth of a child who would have been healthy. Such claims must be distinguished from all claims in respect of the birth of a *disabled* child by the parents (*wrongful birth*) or by the child itself (*wrongful life*). These two claims are different from a routine tort claim for prenatal harm resulting in avoidable injuries (*prenatal injury claim*). In the case of wrongful birth and wrongful life claims, the essence is that if there had been no negligence, *the child would not have been born*: the defendant in these cases did not *cause* the child's disability (which is the '*fault*' of nature), but failed to avert it, while in prenatal injury claims, the child is born injured and alleges that his injury was *caused by* the negligence of another prior to his birth, and therefore seeks damages because, were it not for the defendant's negligence, *he would have existed without injury*.

As already mentioned, wrongful birth and wrongful life both arise from the same circumstances, namely that a physician (or the geneticist or the laboratory) violated the duty of care by conduct falling short of the professional standard of due care. Developments in the field of medical genetics persuaded courts that physicians owe a duty of care, more precisely a duty to warn or to inform parents (or the future child) of genetic risks, and that parents have a right to prevent the birth of children with defects. Liability cases often arise from a doctor's failure to uncover genetic birth defects *in utero* (for instance, when a doctor tells the parents that a prenatal disorder is not genetic in nature, whereas in fact it was a genetic disorder), or from failure to properly interpret the results of a test. But also cases in which a doctor neglects to provide a medical indication for a test, so that as a result no test is performed, or when he refuses a genetic test to parents, when it turns out that there in fact is some medical indication, can lead to liability claims. Finally, insufficient or incorrect information about the unreliability of test results could have deprived the applicant of certain options. Whether or not there is a breach of this duty depends on the standard of care that is to be expected from the doctor, not that of the excellent doctor, but that of a reasonable average doctor of the same specialization, placed in the same circumstances. Moreover it has to be proved that the breach of the duty to warn caused a legally recognized injury. On this particular point there is a large difference between the acceptance of wrongful birth claims and wrongful life claims.

Wrongful birth claims.   In general, *wrongful birth* claims have been awarded in a number of decisions [Bundesgerichtshof, 1997; Conseil d'État (Fr.), 1997; Cour de Cassation (Fr.), 1996, nx 155; Cour de Cassation (Fr.), 1996, nx 156; *Emeh v Kensington and Chelsea and Westminster Area Health Authority* (1984) 3 All ER 1044 (CA); *Thake v Maurice* (1986) 1 All ER 497 (CA)], on the condition that the parents had the *intention* to perform a TOP in the event of an unfavourable diagnosis. Legally, damage is the result of a comparison between the actual situation in which one currently finds oneself and the hypothetical situation in which one would have found oneself had there been no negligent (medical) action. The courts that award the *wrongful birth* claims seem to work on the assumption that, for the parents, the damage consists in the costs of care and education which derive from the handicap. One could seriously doubt the correctness of this opinion: since in principle the child is wanted, the parents cannot claim the normal expenses for care and education, in contrast with *wrongful pregnancy or conception* claims, but only the extra costs deriving from the handicap. Only compensating the extra costs deriving from the handicap would imply that, in jurisprudence, only the handicap is to be considered as damage, as the integral remuneration of the (foreseeable) damage is the rule. Such reasoning, however, is the result of the comparison between handicapped life (actual situation) and normal healthy life. In the comparison the hypothetical situation in the absence of fault is filled-in with 'healthy life', but (i) this was never a possibility in fact and (ii) actually the claim could never be awarded in such a case, since the intention to have *no child* if there had been no fault, is a requirement of admissibility for a *wrongful birth* claim. So in fact the only correct comparison is that between 'handicapped life' and 'non-existence'.

In legal terms, the only damage that can be taken into consideration is the *loss of the chance to undergo an abortion*. Notice that the doctrine of loss of chance is not accepted by all jurisdictions. Germany and the UK (when a doctor's liability is at stake), for instance, do not accept it. In France and Belgium in contrast, the judges have no problem with applying this theory, and in The Netherlands it has only very recently been accepted (Giesen, 1999). If there had been no fault, the parents would *certainly* have retained all possibilities for choice, including the *possibility* to eventually perform a TOP, but it can never be known *for certain* that in the absence of negligence the child would not have been born. The birth of the child is the consequence of many concurrent factors, not the mere result of the fault of the physician, so that the costs of care and education are even a far more indirect consequence. The physician did not *cause* the handicap or disorder: that actually is the 'fault' of nature. In other words, it is never *certain* that the child would not have been born at all in the absence of a fault, so that the birth of the child cannot be retained as a legally certain damage, whereas the loss of a chance to undergo an abortion or to use contraceptives can.

Wrongful life claims.   In the field of *wrongful life* claims, it has usually been stated that there is no damage with regard to the child, since this would constitute a comparison between its actual situation (handicapped life) and its hypothetical situation in the absence of a fault (non-existence). Nobody can, with good reason, make such a comparison, because this would open the way to eugenics [Kennedy and Grubb, 2000. In the UK, wrongful life claims are ruled out by the Congenital Disabilities (civil liability) Act 1976]. Another argument for rejecting these claims is that a fault by the physician did not by itself cause damage to the child, if such damage is taken to be its handicapped life, but that this handicap is a part of the genetic constitution of the child. Nevertheless we are actually talking about the same facts as in *wrongful birth* claims, but here the damage is defined otherwise. It seems that in the case where the parents are the claimants, a comparison is also being made between handicapped life and non-existence. Indeed, if the damage consists in the costs for care and education, then this is the implicit result of a comparison between the extra costs for a handicapped life and non-existence, or with 'healthy life', but this actually never was an option, since the child would suffer in any case from the disorder were it to be born.

Nonetheless, in the literature the possibility of a *wrongful life* claim is nowadays often defended on the grounds that it would be immoral not to compensate a child suffering damage when there is some fault causally connected with that damage. But following the reasoning outlined above, this argument is not acceptable, as there is no causal connection between the physician's negligence and the child's handicap, but only between the fault and the loss of a chance to undergo an abortion. The child has no legitimate interest in this damage, as abortion legislation intends *to protect* unborn life.

Notwithstanding these objections, the French *Cour de Cassation* recently awarded a wrongful life claim [Cour de Cassation (Fr.), 2000, consenting report Sargos, dissenting conclusion Sainte-Rose]. It should be noted that this case did not concern a prenatal *genetic* diagnosis. In this case the child was born with Gregg's syndrome as a result of the mother contracting a rubella infection during pregnancy. The faults committed by the physician and the laboratory, which were never contested before the *Cour de Cassation*, consisted in not properly performing the diagnostic test. To what extent the reasoning set out in this judgement can be applied in cases of prenatal *genetic* testing *for late-onset diseases* is difficult to say, as in such cases the fetus still has a life expectancy of several years without a handicap. However, as this was the first European court to grant a wrongful life claim, and because of the extensive media attention it got, we will discuss it here. In the *Perruche* case of 17 November 2000 the French *Cour de Cassation* decided that 'the faults committed by the physician and the laboratory (. . .) made it impossible for Mrs Perruche to exercise her right to terminate her pregnancy in order to prevent the birth of a handicapped child, so that the latter can claim compensation for the prejudice resulting from those faults.' This key sentence forms the entire decision of the Court, quite brief, not only in comparison with common-law judgements, but also with regard to the social, ethical and legal consequences of this decision.

The report by P. Sargos, however, counsellor of the *Cour de Cassation*, which obviously inspired the Court in its decision, is rather extensive and deals with several issues that arise in this context. The general questions, as the faults were not contested, were the causal connection and the prejudice to the child.

3.4 The causal connection

According to Sargos, one must ask whether, in the absence of the faults, the prejudice could have been prevented. In this case, the child's handicap is the *direct consequence* of the faults committed, as without these faults, there would not have been a handicap. The child would not have been born either in that case, but this consequence has no impact on the causal connection between the fault and the damage, i.e. the handicap. Sargos further argues that the causal connection should not be seen in biological terms of causation, and in doing so the only criterion to decide whether or not to award a *wrongful life* claim can be found in the basic principle of respect for the human person. Following this analysis, and thus accepting a causal connection between fault and handicap, the question of responsibility can be formulated as 'Did the child, born handicapped, suffer a legitimate prejudice, in other words, can it make abstraction of life itself?'

However the Advocate-General J. Sainte-Rose, applying a 'biological' conception of causality, argued in his conclusions that the child's claim and the parents' claim may not be treated similarly: the general rules of liability must be respected, and these demand that there be a causal connection between the fault and the damage, taking account of the fact that not every prejudice can be legitimately compensated. For him, the existence of a *direct* causal connection between the fault of the physician and the damage, in this case the handicap, is problematic as this handicap resulted from an accidental infection. Even in the broadest category of legal causation, i.e. the theory of equivalence, which implies that every fact that was necessary in order to produce the damage is a cause, one could still not claim that there exists a causal connection between the fault and the handicap, as the latter is biological in origin and the fault would never have had an impact on the evolution of the disorder. Saying that the fault is in a causal connection, so that in its absence the damage could have been prevented, would impose on the physician an obligation to ensure in every pregnancy or planned pregnancy the birth of a healthy child.

The physician, therefore, can never be held responsible for causing the handicap; the only damage to which he contributed is the birth of the child, to the extent of having hindered the pregnant woman in choosing for a TOP. But even in that case it is not at all certain that, confronted with an unfavourable diagnosis, the mother actually would have chosen to terminate her pregnancy. The only thing that is certain is that she lost the chance to choose freely whether or not to have a TOP. It is bizarre, therefore, that the child could invoke the certainty that his or her parents would have chosen TOP had they known the diagnosis, as it remains an open question what the mother would ultimately have done. The power to prevent the birth of the child lies with the mother and with no one else.

3.5 Prejudice to the child

According to Sargos, there is a causal connection between the committed faults and the child's handicap. The crucial question for him is to determine whether a child born handicapped suffered a prejudice, as without the faults there would not have been a handicap, but neither would there have been life. Because, in his view, birth and handicap are inseparably linked, the damage of the child (the handicap) necessarily consists at the same time in being born. In other words, the interest of the child not to be handicapped, if we accept the causal connection, in fact consists in the interest not to be born at all, rather than to be born handicapped.

Several authors have criticized the very possibility of a wrongful life claim, because there is no prejudice to the child in being born handicapped as opposed to not being born: deciding otherwise would imply that there is life that is not worth being lived and would form a decisive step towards 'official eugenics'. Furthermore, it is not obvious that one can compare the actual situation of handicapped life with the hypothetical situation of non-existence. How should such damage be evaluated, and is it possible for judges to evaluate such 'prejudice'? And if 'life' constitutes the damage, then 'death' is the absence of damage: death becomes a value more preferable than life.

In addition to these ethical criticisms, Sainte-Rose also points out some practical consequences of the acceptance of such claims. If children can claim damages from physicians for being born handicapped, how long will it take before courts also grant wrongful life claims by children *against their parents*? And there is a risk that allowing such claims will raise the pressure on parents and physicians to minimize the risk of later malpractice claims, so that in cases where there is doubt about the risk of a possible handicap, they would more quickly recommend TOP or more easily comply with a request for prenatal (and preconceptional or preimplantation) genetic diagnosis, even in the absence of a clear medical indication. From that point of view, the possibility of the mother to freely choose whether to terminate the pregnancy might become an obligation, as according to Loisel '*Qui peut et n'empêche, pêche*' (Whoever can prevent, must prevent).

Notwithstanding these critical remarks, the *Cour de Cassation* followed the opinion of Sargos and granted the child's claim. But it is clear that the *Cour de cassation* granted the claim rather as an act of generosity, to permit the child to receive compensation in addition to the aid awarded by the state. As Sargos puts it: 'Where is the real respect for the human person and for life: in the abstract refusal of any compensation, or on the contrary in its admission, that will make it possible for the child to live, at least from a materialistic point of view, in conditions that are more in conformity with human dignity and without being left to the mercies of family, private or public assistance.' The intention of this judgement, then, is certainly praiseworthy, as the insufficiency of the subsidies awarded to handicapped persons has been unanimously denounced. But it can be seriously questioned whether the solution based on civil liability law is the most appropriate way to come to the aid of handicapped persons. As Sainte-Rose argued, this is a question of social law and national solidarity.

This judgement was later on in other cases confirmed by the *Cour de Cassation*, in three decisions of 13 July 2001 and two decisions of 28 November 2001. But we still have not heard the final word on this matter, since on 10 January 2002, the *Assemblée National* adopted a bill (first lecture) *"concerning national solidarity and the compensation of congenital handicaps"*, tending to prohibit wrongful life claims. In its actual version, the bill states that *"no one can claim compensation for the bare fact of his birth, when born handicapped"*. But, at the same time, the bill acknowledges the claim for *wrongful birth* by the parents, but also goes further than that, by adding that the compensation to be paid to parents for the extra expenses deriving from the handicap, relates to the entire life span of the handicapped person (decreased with the amount of the benefits awarded in virtue of national solidarity). As a consequence the compensation does not end, as is normally the case, at the moment the child reaches the age of majority.

4. Concluding remarks

Prenatal testing for late-onset neurological diseases confronts us with some difficult legal questions. Although they cannot be labelled as entirely 'new', the possibility of detecting *in utero* that the child will, as an adult, suffer from a severe neurological disease is an element that 'colours' in a particular way the legal questions that surround prenatal testing in general. The current issue is whether the woman wishing to undergo prenatal testing for a late-onset disease has a sufficient interest in it. Does she have a right to know about a condition for which treatment may become available in the years to come? Does she have the right to request a TOP in those circumstances? Does she have an *obligation* to request a TOP in light of the growing acceptance of wrongful life claims? Does she have an obligation to *undergo* a TOP because she has no interest in knowing the status of the child to be born? These are difficult questions that, given the lack of a specific legal framework, have been answered by taking into account existing legislation (e.g. abortion laws not recognizing the specificity of prenatal testing for a late onset disease) and general principles of law.

References

Andrews, L.B. (1990) The Randolph W. Thrower Symposium. Genetics and the law. Introduction. *Emory Law J.* **39**: 621.

Annas, G.J., Glantz, L.H. and Roche, P.A. (1995) *The Genetic Privacy Act and Commentary.* Health Law Department, University School of Public Health, Boston.

Bompiani, A. (2001) Current regulations on treatment of genetic data in Italy. *Eur. J. Health Law* **8**: 41–50.

Bundesgerichtshof (1997) 4 March 1997. *NJW* 1997, 1638.

Conseil d'État (Fr.) (1997) 14 February 1997. *La Semaine Juridique* 1997, 22828.

Cour de Cassation (Fr.) (1996) 26 March 1996. *Bull. Civ.* 1996, n° 155.

Cour de Cassation (Fr.) (1996) 26 March 1996. *Bull. Civ.* 1996, n° 156.

Cour de Cassation (Fr.) (2000) 17 November 2000. *J.C.P. 2000*, II, 10438, consenting report Sargos, dissenting conclusion Sainte-Rose.

Cavoukian, A. (1995) Confidentiality issues in genetics: the need for privacy and the right not to know. *Law Hum.Genome Rev.* **2**: 55.

Cerezo Mir, J. (1998) *Curso de Derecho Penal Español, II*, 6 edn. Tecnos, Madrid.

Chadwick, R. (1997) The philosophy of the right to know and the right not to know. In: *The Right to Know and the Right Not to Know* (eds R. Chadwick M. Levitt and D. Schicke). Avebury, Aldershot, p. 20.

Danish Council of Ethics (1993) Protection of sensitive personal information. With special reference to genetic data. *Ethics and Mapping of the Human Genome. Fifth Annual Report.* Danish Council of Ethics, Copenhagen, 1993.

De Sola, C. (1994) Privacy and genetic data: situations of conflict (I). *Law Hum.Genome Rev.* **1**: 178–186.

Emeh v Kensington and Chelsea and Westminster Area Health Authority [1984] 3 All ER 1044 (CA).

European Court of Justice (1994) nr. C–404/92 P, 5 October 1994 (X v. Commission), *Jur. H.v.J.* 1994, I–4737, nr. 17.

European Group on Ethics in Science and New Technologies (1996) *Opinion on Ethical Aspects of Prenatal Diagnosis.*

European Parliament and Council (2000) Directive 95/46/EC of 24 October 1995, on the protection of physical persons with regard to the processing of personal data and the free circulation of such data.

Fedder, R.S. (2000) To know or not to know. Legal perspectives on genetic privacy and disclosure of an individual's genetic profile. *J. Legal Med.* **21**: 557.

Giesen, I., (1999) *Bewijslastverdeling bij beroepsaansprakelijkheid.* (Distribution of the burden of proof in case of professional liability) Tjeenk Willink, Deventer.

Grubb, A. (1998) Abortion. In: *Principles of Medical Law* (eds I. Kennedy and A. Grubb). Oxford University Press, Oxford, pp. 629–630.

Guldix, E. (1993–94) De impact van de medische wetenschap en techniek op het personen-en gezinsrecht. (The impact of medical sciences and techniques on family law). *R. W.* **33**: 1123.

Harper, P. and Tyler, A. (1991) Genetic counselling in Huntington's disease. In: *Huntington's Disease* (ed. P. Harper). Saunders, London, p. 354.

Hottois, G. (1999) Información y saber genéticos. *Law Hum.Genome Rev.* **11**: 43.

Kennedy, I. and Grubb, A. (2000) *Medical Law*, 3th edn. Butterworths, London.

International Huntington Association and the World Federation of Neurology (1994) *Guidelines for the Molecular Genetics Predictive Test in Huntington's Disease.*

Malem Seña, J.F. (1995) Privacy and genetic mapping. *Law Hum.Genome Rev.* **2**: 144.

Martinez-Bullé Goyri, V.M. (1995) Genética humana y derecho a la vida privada. *Genética humana y derecho a la intimidad.* Cuaderno del Núcleo de Estudios Interdisciplinarios en Salud y Derechos Humanos, México, Publ. Universidad Autónoma de México.

Nielsen, L. (1996) Genetic testing and privacy: an European perspective. *Law Hum.Genome Rev.* **4**: 65.

Nuffield Council on Bioethics (1993) *Genetic Screening. Ethical Issues.* Nuffield Council on Bioethics, London.

Porn, I. (1997) The meaning of 'rights' in the right to know debate. In: *The Right to Know and the Right Not to Know* (eds R. Chadwick, M. Levitt and D. Schicke). Avebury, Aldershot, p. 37.

Rodota, S. (1990) Le Droit face aux dilèmmes moraux de la vie et de la mort. In: *XXth Colloquy on European Law.* Council of Europe, Strasbourg.

Romeo Casabona, C.M. (1994), Questions de droits de l'homme dans la recherche en génétique médicale. In *Ethique et génétique humaine*, 2e Symposium du Conseil de l'Europe sur la bioéthique, Conseil de l'Europe, Strasbourg.

Roscam Abbing, E.W. and Gevers, J.K.M. (1996) *Voorspellend medisch onderzoek: Mogelijkheden, verwachtingen en toegang. Rechtsbescherming.* (Predictive medical testing: possibilities, expectations and access. Legal protection.) Vereniging voor Gezondheidsrecht, Utrecht.

Roscam Abbing, H. (1995) Genetic information and third party interests: How to find the right balance? *Law Hum. Genome Rev.* **2:** 4–65.

Royal College of Physicians (1991) *Ethical Issues in Clinical Genetics.* Royal College of Physicians, London.

Skene, L. (2001) Testing a fetus for Huntington's disease: is the mother's consent enough? *Med. Today,* 105–107.

Taupitz, J. (1996) Genetic analysis and the right to self-determination in German Civil Law. *Law Hum. Genome Rev.* **4:** 88.

Taupitz, J. (1998) El derecho a no saber en la legislación alemana (I y II). *Law Human Genome Rev.* **8:** 105, **9:** 163 (see on Part I, 109 ff. the foundations of this right; the author conceives it as a 'defence right').

Thake v Maurice [1986] 1 All ER 497 (CA).

World Health Organization (1997) *Proposed International Guidelines on Ethical Issues in Medical Genetics and Genetic Services.* WHO, Geneva.

Yesley, M.S. (1997) Genetic privacy, discrimination, and social policy: challenges and dilemmas. *Microbial Comp. Genomics* **2:** 33.

7

Preimplantation genetic diagnosis for Huntington's disease

Joep P.M.Geraedts and Ingeborg Liebaers

1. Introduction

Soon after the introduction of presymptomatic or predictive testing for Huntington's disease (HD) by DNA, direct prenatal testing for the disorder became available. However, for many couples the combination of prenatal diagnosis with selective abortion is unacceptable because HD is a late-onset disorder and therefore the child carrying the HD mutation might still expect many years of disease-free life.

In this respect, preimplantation genetic diagnosis (PGD) has an advantage over conventional prenatal testing. Couples at risk of the disease, who would like to prevent the transmission of the disease to their offspring, have the option to go through a medically assisted procedure such as *in vitro fertilization* (IVF), with or without intracytoplasmatic sperm injection (ICSI), followed by *in vitro* diagnosis of the resulting embryos after a few days of development. Only disease-free embryos are transferred to the uterus and therefore couples are not faced with a difficult decision about pregnancy termination. Over the past 10 years, PGD has become available for most of the monogenic and chromosomal disorders for which prenatal testing is available. Patients who prefer PGD over prenatal diagnosis and selective abortion may do so because the latter option conflicts with their fundamental beliefs. They also may select PGD after having one or more conventional prenatal diagnoses with unsuccessful outcomes. Finally, they may opt for PGD because they require medically assisted reproduction (IVF or ICSI) anyway due to infertility.

The main disadvantage of PGD is the low success rate of obtaining a pregnancy, a fact that is substantially influenced by the number of oocytes that can be harvested, and those remaining for transfer after fertilization, biopsy and diagnosis. In a dominant disorder such as HD, the potential number of replaceable embryos is on average reduced by 50%. Other disadvantages are the complexity and psychological distress of the IVF procedure and the medicalization of reproduction.

2. The preimplantation genetic diagnosis procedure

Potential parents referred for PGD are thoroughly evaluated genetically and clinically. Inclusion or exclusion criteria may vary according to the centre performing the test and the disease involved. Genetic evaluation depends on the method of analysis applied (see below). The evaluation of the reproductive file consists of the reproductive history of the couple; a gynaecological examination of the wife; blood tests of the female partner including at least oestradiol, luteinizing hormone (LH) and follicle-stimulating hormone (FSH) between day 2 and day 6 of the cycle, a screening for infectious diseases and a karyotype. Moreover, a vaginal ultrasound to examine the pelvic structures and a mock transfer are performed. For the male partner a sperm analysis and blood tests including a screening for infectious diseases and a karyotype are done. More tests are performed if indicated.

The DNA of both parents is studied for information regarding the normal alleles of the HD gene. At intake special attention is paid to the presence of symptoms indicating signs of onset of HD. In case minor symptoms are noticed a further discussion on the progression of the disease takes place in order to evaluate the couple's view on the future. The limited experience to date does not allow the drawing of any conclusions or proposing strict guidelines concerning the exclusion or inclusion of couples requesting PGD.

Finally the informed consent is signed (*Fig. 1*).

PGD takes place between fertilization and implantation, but in most cases on the third day of early embryonic development. To obtain access to this early development stage, IVF with or without ICSI is necessary, although the women undergoing this treatment are usually normally fertile. ICSI is preferred over conventional IVF in monogenic disorders requiring DNA diagnosis to prevent contamination from sperm still attached to the zona pellucida. After hormonal stimulation on average about 10 oocytes are obtained of which 6 or 7 become fertilized after the medically assisted procedure. The sperm is produced by masturbation in the laboratory immediately preceding IVF. On the third day post insemination one or two blastomeres are biopsied from embryos that have reached about the eight-cell stage. The DNA is then amplified using PCR methodology. Although technically more difficult, the detection method at the single cell level is principally that applied to other tissues, although working with blastomeres has specific difficulties including lysis, multinucleation and allele dropout (Pickering and Muggleton-Harris, 1995). Allele dropout means that just one of the two alleles under study is (selectively) amplified. Other diagnostic problems are caused by embryonic mosaicism or contamination. For these reasons it is advisable to diagnose two cells. Only those embryos in which both cells have been shown to be free of the disease would then be considered unaffected and used for transfer to the uterus or cryopreservation for transfer at

What is preimplantation genetic diagnosis (PGD)?

1. Preimplantation genetic diagnosis is a very new, still experimental technique, which involves detecting an underlying genetic defect by analysing embryos, obtained through in vitro fertilisation (IVF).
2. Up to June 1999, a few hundred children were born world-wide after PGD.
3. During the IVF treatment there is a small risk for hyperstimulation (= liquid in the abdomen), sometimes necessitating hospitalisation.
4. One should not have unprotected sex 1 week before and 1 week after oocyte retrieval.
5. The stimulation cycle will be cancelled when less than 9 follicles (oocytes) are seen at ultrasound.
6. After transfer the chance for pregnancy and birth is expected to be 20%.
7. There is a small risk of misdiagnosis, estimated to be about 1% to 5%. This is why a control chorionic villus sampling or amniocentesis are recommended.
8. Affected embryos will be further analysed and thus destroyed.
9. "Unaffected" embryos will be frozen (if possible) and *can* be replaced, later on.
10. We are fully and extensively informed about the procedure, through several consultations which are summarised in this text.

Read and approved:

Name: .... Name: ....

Date: .... Date: ....

Signature: Signature:

Figure 1. Informed consent for preimplantation genetic diagnosis as used in Brussels.

a later date. A maximum of two unaffected embryos are transferred to the uterus. Human chorionic gonadotrophin (hCG) is determined at day 12. If a pregnancy is established an ultrasound examination at 7 weeks is performed to study fetal heartbeat. Couples positive at this stage are advised to undergo pre-natal diagnosis by chorionic villus sampling or amniocentesis because of the experimental nature of the PGD procedure. The success rate of PGD is expressed as the percentage of babies delivered per cycle and per transfer. Furthermore, if possible and applicable, the following parameters are recorded: hormonal stimulation cycles cancelled, misdiagnoses, pregnancy complications and health of the baby at birth and at 2 years of age (including congenital malformations).

3. Experience with preimplantation genetic diagnosis

In 1997, the European Society for Human Reproduction and Embryology (ESHRE) PGD Consortium was formed as part of the ESHRE Special Interest Group on Reproductive Genetics. The active member centres of this PGD Consortium are situated in the following countries: Australia, Belgium, Denmark, France, Greece, Italy, Korea, The Netherlands, Spain, Sweden, Taiwan, UK and USA. They represent the majority of activities in the field of PGD in the world.

Here we describe PGD in general. PGD of HD is treated in Section 5. The prospective and retrospective collection of data on availability, accuracy, reliability and effectiveness of PGD has been one of the major aims of the ESHRE PGD Consortium. In December 1999, the first PGD Consortium report was published discussing referrals on 323 couples, 392 PGD cycles and 82 pregnancies (ESHRE PGD-Consortium, 1999). In the second data collection round, contributing centres were asked to send in data from their PGD activities before this date, as well as from 1 October 1998 to 1 May 2000, in order to have an as complete as possible overview of PGD practices in these centres. In total referral data have been obtained from 886 couples. Patients were referred for PGD because of sexing for X-linked disease, translocations and other structural chromosome abnormalities as well as monogenic diseases. The most frequently referred Mendelian disorders remain constant over the years: cystic fibrosis, thalassaemia and spinal muscular atrophy as autosomal recessive diseases; myotonic dystrophy, HD and Charcot-Marie-Tooth disease as autosomal dominant and Duchenne's muscular dystrophy, Fragile-X syndrome and haemophilia as X-linked disorders.

The vast majority of couples have had one or more pregnancies prior to PGD. However, healthy children have been born in fewer than 25% of them. More than a quarter of all couples have one or more affected children. The proportion of couples having experienced one or more spontaneous abortions or terminations of pregnancy after prenatal diagnosis amount to 27.4 and 22.1% respectively.

This is reflected in the reasons for PGD. The most important reason is genetic risk and objection to termination of pregnancy (44%). The group having experienced termination after prenatal diagnosis is smaller (28%). In almost one-third of the cases (29%) the genetic indication was combined with sub- or infertility, which made IVF with or without ICSI necessary.

Cycle data were obtained on 1319 cycles.

PCR-based diagnoses were performed for a variety of autosomal recessive and dominant disorders and for sexing or specific diagnosis for X-linked diseases. For the PCR diagnosis, 385 cycles reached oocyte retrieval. As mentioned earlier, it is well documented that for PCR diagnosis fertilization should be achieved by ICSI to reduce the risk of contamination from sperm embedded in the zona pellucida, but IVF was used in 35 cycles. A successful PCR diagnosis was obtained in 81% of embryos successfully biopsied, and 55% were diagnosed as transferable.

FISH-based diagnoses were performed in couples at risk for X-linked disease to determine the sex of the embryos and in patients carrying Robertsonian and reciprocal translocations.

In total, pregnancy data were obtained on 163 pregnancies. The high rate of multiple pregnancies (31%) was in contrast to the moderate pregnancy rate per cycle (16.5%). As far as complications of pregnancy are concerned it is clear that an important proportion of these (preterm labour, premature rupture of membranes) originated from multiple pregnancies. Not much difference was noted between the PGD children group at birth and a control group born after 'regular' ICSI, described by Bonduelle et al. (1999). In both series 52 and 54%

were singletons, 46 and 41% were twins and 2 and 5% were triplets. Parameters such as birth weight were very similar: singletons weighed 3206 and 3220 g and twins weighed 2344 and 2421 g, respectively. Birth length and head circumference were equally similar. When the definition of major malformation (a malformation that generally causes functional impairment or requires surgical correction) was applied, a rate of 3/130 (bilateral clubfoot, exencephaly and chylothorax) or 2.3% was obtained in the PGD group. Again, this is very close to the 2.9% obtained by Bonduelle *et al.* (1999). Although concerning small numbers as yet, an important message of the ESHRE PGD Consortium is that PGD babies are not exposed to greater risks of neonatal problems or malformation than ICSI babies, which in turn do not display more malformations than naturally conceived children.

Four misdiagnoses for monogenetic diseases were reported, after prenatal diagnosis, which is advised for confirmation of this still experimental procedure. In two of these cases the pregnancies were terminated. It is very important to note that all cases of misdiagnosis occurred after the use of PCR. One of these misdiagnoses was probably due to contamination. For the other three no explanation was given or available, although it would be interesting to know why these misdiagnoses occurred in order to prevent such events in the future, possibly through guidelines issued by the PGD Consortium. These data have been published recently (ESHRE-PGD Consortium, 2000).

4. Availability of preimplantation genetic diagnosis

Since the first report on clinically applied PGD in 1990 by Handyside and colleagues in the UK, the number of centres involved in PGD has increased year by year. The availability of PGD in Europe was summarized by Viville and Pergament in 1998. In *Table 1* we have tried to give an overview representing the situation in November 2000. It is based on information available within the ESHRE PGD Consortium and completed through personal communications

Table 1. The availability of preimplantation genetic diagnosis in Europe

Country	PGD regulated by law	PGD permitted	Number of centres
Austria	+	−	0
Belgium	−	+	3
Denmark	+	+	1
Finland	+	+	0
France	+	+	3
Germany	+	?	0
Greece	−	+	1
Italy	−	+	2
Norway	+	+	0
Spain	+	+	2
Sweden	+	+	2
The Netherlands	−	+	1
UK	+	+	4

of many European colleagues from various countries. It shows that a division can be seen between countries with and without legislation regulating PGD. Some of the countries with legislation have a law allowing PGD (UK, Spain) while it is clear that PGD is not allowed in others (Austria). In Germany the state of affairs is unclear as the law can be interpreted in different ways. In countries without legislation PGD is sometimes allowed under the guidance of a national authority. Belgium, Greece, Italy and The Netherlands are examples of this. Finally, the situation in Norway is such that PGD is allowed, but not for HD and in any case not done for other diseases either.

5. Preimplantation genetic diagnosis for Huntington's disease

As in prenatal diagnosis, PGD for HD is possible via direct 'CAG' testing and indirect exclusion testing. The latter method is based on the indirect detection of alleles from the affected grandparent by a marker system linked to the HD gene. Finally, PGD is also possible via so-called non-disclosure testing. This highly controversial procedure entails direct testing of the expanded repeat on the embryos without knowing the disease status of the proband at risk.

5.1 Direct testing

PGD through direct CAG-repeat testing was first reported by Sermon *et al.* (1998). This method was originally based on the amplification and detection of the non-expanded 'healthy' alleles of both partners. The first PGD cycles were only performed for couples that were 100% informative, which means that the non-expanded allele of the affected parent needed to be different from both alleles of the non-affected parent. Later as the experience with the assay rose and the expanded allele of the carrier parent to be was always observed, 50% informative couples were also accepted for PGD.

5.2 Preimplantation genetic diagnosis exclusion testing

Predictive testing for adults at risk was originally proposed as a method for prenatal diagnosis by Harper and Sarfarazi (1985). It allows a parent with a 50% risk of having HD to have children with a low risk of having HD.

Originally, exclusion testing was a procedure offering the possibility of prenatal diagnosis to couples for whom an informative predictive test result based on linked markers was unavailable because of an incomplete pedigree. Later on, at-risk persons who, on the one hand, did not want to know their own carrier status but who, on the other hand, did not want to possibly transmit the disease, started to make use of this exclusion testing procedure. The principle of the test is to analyse chorionic villi of a fetus at risk for the presence or absence of one of the chromosomes 4 of the affected grandparent by the use of markers linked to the HD locus and without revealing the carrier status of the at-risk parent to be. The final aim of the test is to terminate the pregnancy if one of the chromosomes 4 of the affected grandparent is transmitted resulting in a 50% risk to the fetus to develop HD later in life. However, since on average half of the aborted fetuses will not carry the HD allele and would therefore not have developed the disease, it may be argued that abortion in these cases is unethical or at least too much of a burden. PGD through exclusion testing may, therefore, be a better alternative. If linked DNA markers are used to determine whether the HD allele which has been passed to the embryo from the at-risk parent originated from the affected or unaffected grandparent and if the linkage analysis indicates inheritance from the grandparent with HD, the embryo shares the same 50% risk of being affected with HD as the intervening parent. Once detected, these embryos will be excluded for transfer notwithstanding that only half of these embryos will contain the affected allele. Although the number of embryos available for transfer is no fewer than if direct testing is used because in both instances half of the embryos may be unsuitable for transfer, exclusion PGD is considered ethically dubious by some because of the discarding of normal embryos. However, it must be remembered that this approach is not unique as it is directly analogous to the use of PGD by FISH to detect gender in sex-linked disorders in which half of the embryos selected against may not carry the disorder (Braude *et al.*, 1998).

5.3 Non-disclosure preimplantation genetic diagnosis

Most parents do not wish to pass on the HD gene mutation to their children, but may not themselves be prepared to undergo presymptomatic testing and learn about their own genetic status. Therefore, many at-risk individuals with a family history of HD would prefer a method of genetic diagnosis that would assure them that they can have children unaffected with HD without revealing their own genetic status (non-disclosing). For non-disclosure PGD, the couples would be told only that fertilization had occurred, that embryos were formed and tested, and that only embryos that are apparently free of the disease were transferred to the uterus. The parents would not be given any information that might provide a basis for inferring whether any embryos with HD were ever identified (Schulman *et al.*, 1996). Couples undergoing non-disclosing PGD are aware of the possibility that they will undergo IVF and may not be at-risk for HD, but accept this as necessary to maintain their choice of non-disclosure of their HD risk. There are a number of problems related to this type of diagnosis. First of all it is difficult to keep the test results and the embryological information secret. There are many people involved in the IVF/ICSI treatment and the PGD procedure: clinical geneticists, gynaecologists, nurses, secretarial personnel, embryologists, technicians, molecular geneticists, etc. It will be extremely difficult not to reveal some information on the basis of which the couple might get an idea of the carrier status. Furthermore, if no embryos are available for transfer, the couple might conclude that all of them were affected. However, if no affected embryos are diagnosed in a large cohort, it might be unnecessary to offer a second treatment cycle.

6. Experience with preimplantation genetic diagnosis for Huntington's disease

6.1 Brussels

The first requests for PGD of HD date back to 1995. In 1998 the first diagnostic method for direct testing was ready to be applied in the clinic (Sermon *et al.*, 1998).

Between 1995 and 2000, 32 couples had contacted the clinic to inquire about PGD for HD. Twenty-eight couples asked for direct testing and four asked for exclusion testing. Of these 24 couples were informative or semi-informative for the healthy/expanded CAG repeats and therefore eligible for PGD. Only two of the four couples interested in exclusion testing attended the clinic and only in one couple were informative markers identified and used in a PCR assay at the single cell level in order to offer PGD.

Exclusion testing was considered to be an acceptable alternative to direct testing for couples at risk who did not want presymptomatic testing but who wanted to avoid the transmission of the disease to their offspring. As well for the direct test as for the exclusion test, two cells from eight-cell embryos were biopsied and analysed. Only embryos of which both cells displayed the same result, namely only carrying 'healthy' CAG repeats in case of direct testing or only carrying non at-risk linked markers in exclusion testing, were transferred into the uterus.

PGD was performed in 16 couples from the following countries: Belgium (7), France (1), Germany (3), Ireland (1), Italy (1) and United Kingdom (3). In 15 couples direct testing was done and in 1 couple (2 cycles) exclusion testing.

The *at-risk* persons were equally divided over the sexes: in eight cases each the male partner and the female partner were the affected parent.

The reasons for having PGD were as follows: objection to abortion (7); previous termination (7) and infertility (2). The reproductive history of these couples are summarized in *Tables 2–4*.

The mean maternal age was 30 years (range 21–34). A total of 30 cycles was started. In 27 of these 1 or 2 embryos were transferred. Seven patients had one PGD treatment cycle and two became pregnant; five patients had two cycles but no pregnancy; three patients had three cycles and two became pregnant; one patient had four cycles before becoming pregnant. The ongoing pregnancy

Table 2. Patient history/reason for preimplantation genetic diagnosis: objection to abortion

1. Three PGDs, pregnant, no CVS, healthy baby, will come back for second child
2. Two PGDs, not pregnant, undecided about next cycle (recent previous cycle)
3. Two PGDs, not pregnant, undecided about next cycle (recent previous cycle)
4. Two PGDs, not pregnant, pause
5. One PGD, not pregnant, undecided about next cycle (cost)
6. One PGD, not pregnant
7. One PGD, pregnant

Table 3. Patient history/reason for PGD: Previous terminations

1. $G_3P_1A_2$; two PGDs, not pregnant; $G_4P_1A_3$; one PGD, not pregnant, undecided about next cycle (recent previous cycle)
2. $G_5P_0A_4$; four PGDs; pregnant, CVS, healthy baby
3. $G_2P_0A_2$; one PGD, not pregnant; $G_3P_0A_3$; baby born post CVS (no PGD)
4. $G_1P_0A_1$; three PGDs; pregnant, CVS?
5. $G_3P_1A_2$; one PGD, not pregnant; $G_4P_1A_3$; baby born post CVS (no PGD)
6. $G_1P_0A_1$; one PGD; not pregnant, next cycle planned
7. $G_2P_0A_2$; two PGDs; not pregnant, next cycle planned

rate was 17% per started PGD cycle, 18.5% per embryo transfer and 31% per patient. In total three babies were born and two pregnancies were ongoing after PGD. A total of 183 embryos were biopsied. In 30 (17%) no diagnosis was obtained. Of the 153 embryos diagnosed 80 (55%) were affected and the remaining 73 (48%) were unaffected.

6.2 Maastricht

When PGD was started in Maastricht in 1995, the KEMO, a provisional central ethical review board, held the view that the first clinical application of PGD needed to be restricted to severe conditions for which no treatment was available because of the burden, the uncertainties and the risks of this still experimental procedure. It was decided to start with diagnosis of some X-linked disorders such as Duchenne's muscular dystrophy and fragile-X syndrome, cystic fibrosis and spinal muscular atrophy and not to include HD in the list of diagnoses offered, because of the late onset of the disease.

At the end of 1998 a Health Council Committee had the opinion that PGD had been introduced judiciously in The Netherlands. Furthermore, it was recommended that the inclusion and exclusion criteria needed not to be stricter than those used for prenatal diagnosis with the exception of aneuploidy screening for risks related to advanced maternal age such as trisomy 21. Therefore, it was decided to offer PGD for HD and to start with direct testing of embryos from known disease gene carriers and their partners and not to offer the alternatives of non-disclosure or exclusion testing.

The first group to be offered direct testing needed to fulfil the following criteria: (i) the couple is fully informative for the normal CAG repeats, (ii) no allele is in the 'grey zone' (35–39 repeats), (iii) There are no contraindications for IVF/ICSI, and (iv) there are no obvious signs of the disease. The direct testing is based on the analysis of the 'healthy' CAG repeats as well as the expanded ones as described by Sermon *et al.* (1998).

Table 4. Patient history/reason for preimplantation genetic diagnosis: fertility problem

1. $G_4P_1A_3 \rightarrow$ (post fertility treatment); one PGD; pregnant, CVS, healthy baby
2. $G_0P_0A_0$ (male azoospermic); two PGDs; not pregnant

In total, 32 couples have been referred. In 16 cases the female was gene carrier and in 15 the male partner. One male was at risk but did not want to know his carrier status. The obstetric histories showed no pregnancies in 16 couples, previous prenatal diagnosis and termination of pregnancy in 13 and normal offspring in 2 couples only. Three couples had a principal objection to prenatal diagnosis (if no PGD, no children). The couple with the male at risk requested non-disclosure or exclusion testing, which was refused. One prospective parent was symptomatic, for which reason the couple could not be helped. One couple was unsuitable for IVF. Three couples were not informative for the normal alleles. In two cases there was a spontaneous pregnancy before PGD was performed. Four couples refrained from treatment and two others postponed it. From the 18 remaining couples the treatment of 9 has started. In total 16 cycles resulted in 5 pregnancies (1 biochemical, 1 ongoing and 3 delivered). Of the 102 embryos examined, 49 were unaffected, 50 affected and in 3 there was no diagnosis.

6.3 Other centres in Europe

From the ESHRE PGD Consortium database it is known that besides the centres in Brussels and Maastricht only one other centre in Europe is offering PGD for HD. This is namely Professor Braude's Division of Women's and Children's Health from the St. Thomas' Hospital in London, UK. Up to the end of the year 2000 there were 35 referrals, 10 of which were for exclusion testing. The latter is not offered due to the many ethical, practical and clinical problems (Braude *et al.* 1998). The centre is waiting for permission from the Human Fertilization and Embryology Authority to start the clinical PGD procedure with direct testing in couples known to be at risk after predictive testing.

6.4 The USA: Fairfax

As far as we know, the Genetics & IVF Group at Fairfax is the only centre in the USA helping individuals at-risk for HD, who do not wish to pass on the gene for HD to their children, but may not be prepared themselves to undergo presymptomatic testing and learn their genetic status. These involved couples where one partner was at 50% risk for HD. After extensive counselling and informed consent 10 couples underwent 13 IVF and 2 frozen embryo transfer cycles in a programme for non-disclosing PGD for HD. In 11 cycles embryos determined to be free of HD were transferred resulting in 5 clinical pregnancies. Both HD mutation carrier and non-carrier couples successfully achieved pregnancy.

One set of twins and a singleton pregnancy have delivered and two other pregnancies are ongoing. One pregnancy resulted in a first trimester loss. These authors believe that non-disclosing PGD offers an important new reproductive alternative for individuals faced with the prospect of a fatal neurodegenerative disorder and a desire to have healthy children. The Fairfax group has reported the successful implementation of such a non-disclosing PGD programme at their institute. They claim to have demonstrated that with meticulous attention to confidentiality, careful genetic counselling and fully informed consent, one can successfully assist at-risk couples who do not want predictive testing to have their own biological children free of HD (Stern *et al.*, 2000).

7. Discussion

Many couples referred for PGD have objections to termination of pregnancy after prenatal diagnosis and it seems that for a number of them PGD is the only option which is acceptable. Although the couples are normally fertile, the pregnancy rates are not yet in agreement with a fertile population. Most probably this results mainly from the reduction of the number of embryos available for transfer and, to a lesser extent, from increased parental ages. Misdiagnosis has not been reported yet. In general, there is no evidence for an increase of congenital abnormalities other than from the increased rate of multiple pregnancies. It seems that the practice of PGD for HD is becoming more and more established and it is to be expected that the number of centres offering this procedure will slowly but steadily increase. (Note added in proof: In 2001 there were reports of the introduction of PGD in Sydney, Melbourne and Chicago.)

PGD based on direct testing with disclosure will probably be the first and maybe the only choice for most centres. PGD based on direct testing without disclosure may be or become a first choice for many couples but the practical application may remain problematic (Braude *et al.*, 1998). However, the first results in Fairfax seem promising (Stern *et al.*, 2000). PGD based on exclusion testing may develop with time by working out single cell multiplex PCR procedures for a panel of linked markers from which the informative ones can be chosen for each requesting couple. In these cases, however, a linkage analysis in the family has to be performed before the PGD procedure can be offered.

From a recent overview on prenatal diagnosis of HD in The Netherlands it can be seen that yearly on average about 12 direct tests and 4 exclusion tests are carried out for the country as a whole (Maat-Kievit *et al.*, 1999). From these data it can be concluded that PGD is certainly an option for a relatively high number of HD gene carriers as the number of patients referred for PGD is in the same order of magnitude as the number of patients referred for prenatal diagnosis. In this respect PGD for HD differs from PGD for other diseases. PGD of HD poses a specific dilemma, which does not exist in prenatal diagnosis. The presence of the disease in and finally the loss of one of the parents is predictable although the decrease in mental and physical function may be variable. This has implications for any child born into the relationship and for any existing children. It is of particular importance in the UK where it is a legal requirement under terms of the Human Fertilization and Embryology Act (1990) to take into account the welfare of any child born as a result of assisted conception before offering treatment. However, the alternative is to leave it up to the parents to establish a pregnancy and then to do prenatal diagnosis, eventually followed by selective abortion. Therefore, the outcome of both procedures might eventually be identical although the price that has been paid is different (Chapter 9).

Acknowledgements

We wish to thank the following colleagues in Brussels: Karen Sermon, Paul Devroey, Andre Van Steirteghem and many co-workers of the Centre for Medical Genetics and Centre for Reproductive Medicine. In Maastricht: Jos Dreesen, Hans Evers, Christine de Die, John Dumoulin and all other members of the PGD Working Group. Finally, we would like to express our gratitude to Cees Varkevisser and Gerrit Dommerholt for their cooperation as representatives of the Dutch Huntington Society.

References

Bonduelle, M., Camus, M., De Vos, A., et al. (1999) Seven years of intracytoplasmic sperm injection and follow-up of 1987 subsequent children. *Hum. Reprod.* **14 (Suppl. 1):** 243–264.

Braude, P.R., De Wert, G.M., Evers-Kiebooms, G., Pettigrew, R.A. and Geraedts, J.P. (1998) Non-disclosure preimplantation diagnosis for Huntington's disease: practical and ethical dilemmas. *Prenatal. Diag.* **18:** 1422–1426.

ESHRE PGD Consortium Steering Committee (1999) ESHRE Preimplantation Genetic Diagnosis (PGD) Consortium: preliminary assessment of data from January 1997 to September 1998. *Hum. Reprod.* **14:** 3138–3148.

ESHRE PGD Consortium Steering Committee (2000) ESHRE Preimplantation Genetic Diagnosis (PGD) Consortium: data collection II (May 2000). *Hum. Reprod.* **15:** 2673–2683.

Handyside, A.H., Kontogianni, E.H., Hardy, K. and Winston, R.M.L. (1990) Pregnancies from biopsied human preimplantation embryos sexed by Y-specific DNA amplification. *Nature* **344:** 768–770.

Harper, P.S. and Sarfarazi, M. (1985) Genetic prediction and family structure in Huntington's chorea. *BMJ* **290:** 1929–1931.

Maat-Kievit, A., Vegter-van der Vlis, M., Zoeteweij, M., et al. (1999) Experience in prenatal testing for Huntington's disease in the Netherlands: procedures, results and guidelines (1987–1997). *Prenatal Diag.* **19:** 450–457.

Pickering, S.J. and Muggleton-Harris, A.L. (1995) Reliability and accuracy of polymerase chain reaction amplification of two unique target sequences from biopsies of cleavage-stage and blastocyst-stage human embryos. *Molec. Hum. Reprod.* **10:** 1021–1029.

Schulman, J.D., Black, S.H., Handyside, A. and Nance, W.E. (1996) Preimplantation genetic testing for Huntington disease and certain other dominantly inherited disorders. *Clin. Genet.* **49:** 57–58.

Sermon, K., Goossens, V., Seneca, S., et al. (1998) Preimplantation diagnosis for Huntington's disease (HD): clinical application and analysis of the HD expansion in affected embryos. *Prenatal Diag.* **18:** 1427–1436.

Stern, H.J., Harton, G.L., Sisson, S.L. et al. (2000) Non-disclosing preimplantation genetic diagnosis for Huntington disease. *Am. J. Hum. Genet.* **67 (Suppl. 2):** 42.

Viville, S. and Pergament, D. (1998) Results of a survey of the legal status and attitudes towards preimplantation genetic diagnosis conducted in 13 different countries. *Prenatal Diagn.* **18:** 1374–1380.

8

Case histories about preimplantation genetic diagnosis

Christine de Die and Nathalie Heurckmans

1. Introduction

Carriers of the Huntington's disease (HD) gene and their spouses may be strongly motivated not to pass on the mutated gene to their offspring. Underlying reasons expressed by future parents are that they do not want their future children to be faced with the same difficult choices as they have to now make and feelings of guilt towards offspring if they pass on the gene despite being fully aware of the risk. Also, they realize that they are the first generation to know of the hereditary nature of the disease and that nowadays realistic methods are available to 'stop' the disease, not only for their own children but also for all future generations. One of our patients expressed his feelings as follows: 'My wife and I feel it as our duty to ban the disease from the family'.

In practice, a minority of known gene carriers chooses prenatal testing and eventual selective termination of pregnancy (Maat-Kieviet *et al.*, 1999). This low uptake for prenatal testing can be explained in part by the fact that almost half of the applicants for predictive testing already have offspring. Other possible reasons for this low uptake are the fear of being unable to cope with an unfavourable test result, resulting in a termination of pregnancy or the risk of the prenatal test itself. Furthermore, it might be explained by ethical reservations about selective abortion for a late-onset disorder, denial, minimalization or hope for a cure for the disease in the future (Maat-Kieviet *et al.*, 2000).

Since 1998, preimplantation genetic diagnosis (PGD) has been an alternative to prenatal testing. PGD may have advantages and disadvantages compared with prenatal testing. The main advantage of PGD is the avoidance of termination of pregnancy in case of an abnormal result. However, PGD has still to be regarded as an experimental procedure with largely unknown (long-term) risks for mothers and their children. The emotional and social burden of PGD,

Prenatal Testing for Late-Onset Neurogenetic Diseases, edited by G. Evers-Kiebooms,
M. W. Zoeteweij and P. S. Harper
©2002 BIOS Scientific Publishers Ltd, Oxford

compared with prenatal testing, may differ for each couple depending on their previous history, their personal circumstances and their moral views.

PGD is offered in genetic centres in Brussels and Maastricht, using direct testing of the expanded CAG repeat in embryos from known gene carriers and their partners (Sermon *et al.*, 1998). For at-risk persons, who do not want to know their disease status, exclusion testing with linked markers is available in Brussels. It was decided not to offer non-disclosure testing in the first series, on the basis of expected practical and technical problems, such as the assurance of absolute secrecy in the *in vitro* fertilization (IVF) procedure (Braude *et al.*, 1998).

We present three couples at risk for offspring with HD who applied for PGD, explore their current situation and discuss their considerations when choosing PGD. The chapter ends with some ethical reflections regarding PGD for late-onset disorders and the acceptability of PGD for individuals who already show signs or symptoms of HD.

2. Case histories

2.1 Case 1

Intake.   In April 2000, Mr B. (32 years old) and Mrs B. (28 years old) visited our centre requesting information on PGD for HD. Mrs B. carries the Huntington's mutation. Her mother is symptomatic. Mrs B. runs a drugstore and Mr B. is an IT professional.

Family of origin of Mrs B.   The mother of Mrs B. showed the first symptoms of HD at 49 years in 1988. Soon thereafter the diagnosis was confirmed. Mrs B. was 16 years old at that time. The grandmother of Mrs B. died earlier from the same disease. Mrs B. has two sisters who were not tested (yet). One has one boy and the other is married but has no children (yet). Huntington's disease had never been mentioned in the family. Mrs B. requested presymptomatic testing at 18 years. She was finally tested at 21 years and found to be carrier of the mutation. Mrs B. was still single when she was tested but she wanted to know her status in view of later children. The fact that her mother had the disease as well as the fact that she was tested positively was a very traumatic experience for her: 'If I become as difficult as my mother I will put an end to my life'. All her dreams were falling apart. She felt isolated and her self-image became negatively coloured. Today, 7 years after the test result, she still experiences her test result as very traumatic. 'I was sentenced to life imprisonment'. As a consequence of these feelings Mrs B. no longer engaged in social contact. She was advised to seek professional help, i.e. relation therapy and individual therapy. She rejected this proposal because she experienced this as another personal failure.

Her mother is still alive and suffers mainly from behavioural problems and sapped Mrs B.'s strength in a psychological way by saying 'You are worth nothing, you are incapable, you can not have children', as well as in a physical way (abuse). Mrs B. never mentioned her father. Within the family these 'things' were never discussed. Everyone suffered and dealt with it in his own way. She had two important goals in her life: finding a husband and having healthy children. She hoped, by succeeding, to increase her self-esteem. Without children she would consider her life to be not worth living.

Relation.   After a 3-year relationship Mrs B. married her husband (in May 1999). For Mrs B. marriage was a very important event, as it reassured her that Mr B. would not leave her. Until the day of the wedding she was expecting him to say that he did not want to marry a person who was a carrier of HD. She informed her husband-to-be about her carrier status when they met for the first time in order to avoid losing him later on. Mr B. is an introvert but says that he realizes very well what HD is. He has observed his mother-in-law's behaviour and worries about his wife's future behaviour. He never mentioned any particular aspects of his fear.

Family of origin of Mr B.   The family of Mr B. knows about the occurrence of HD in their daughter-in-law's family because both families live in the same small village. In that village people talked about 'the family with the strange mother'. Not one of his close relatives knew, however, that Mrs B. had tested positive for HD. Mr B. was afraid that if he told them his family would discourage him from marrying her. He felt mainly that his mother wanted to protect him from life's burdens.

History.   In January 1999, Mrs B. became spontaneously pregnant. The couple was not yet married and both still lived with their parents. This unexpected pregnancy was very disturbing for both of them. They felt guilty for religious reasons but Mrs B. was also happy with the event, as having a child was very important to her. However, they were worried that the fetus would be affected. A chorionic villus sampling, performed at 10 weeks, showed that the fetus was affected and the pregnancy was terminated. Only Mrs B.'s two sisters were informed. No one else, either from Mrs B.'s family or from Mr B.'s family knew about the pregnancy. This secrecy about the prenatal test is understandable. Many tested persons keep their prenatal test secret and do not tell anyone about a termination, probably because of fear of reactions from others. Mrs B. experienced the termination of the pregnancy as difficult and she felt very guilty about it. She again experienced this as a failure: 'I feel as I am not able to conceive healthy children'. She refused to speak about the pain she felt or about the support or the lack of support she got from professionals or from others.

In April 2000, Mr and Mrs B. visited our center for the first time. Mrs B. wanted to have a healthy child as soon as possible, certainly before the age of 30 years. Within that scenario she expected to become symptomatic when the child was 10–15 years old. She wanted the child to be not older than 15 years when she showed the first symptoms. This was related to the fact that she was 16 years old when her mother became ill and this experience had been very traumatic for her: like all adolescents she was searching for herself. This process became difficult on seeing her mother on the decline. She believed that younger children (less than 15 years) would have fewer problems coping with this disease.

The PGD procedure was explained to them and 3 months later they decided to go ahead with PGD although Mrs B.'s expectations were rather negative. It was mainly the fact that a control chorionic villus sampling after PGD was recommended that bothered Mrs B. but she could not really explain why. This can probably be explained by fear of a termination at the last minute.

Mr and Mrs B. are both Catholic and very religious. They say that religion is of great help to them: 'Since God made them suffer a lot already their hope was that he would now accept their choice to have PGD in order to alleviate their suffering'. The main advantage of PGD to them was that they did not have to make a decision concerning the termination of pregnancy. The disadvantage was the medicalization of conception, the lack of romanticism and the fact that so many people/physicians were going to be involved. Mr B. was rather optimistic and thought that the procedure would be successful and lead to a pregnancy. Mrs B. was rather pessimistic: 'I am always unlucky, why should I be lucky this time?'. Adoption or the use of donor gametes was not an option for them. They considered the lack of a genetic link as negative. Parenthood was related more to a genetic link than to an educational alliance for them. In July 2000, they had their first PGD treatment. Hormonal stimulation to prepare for PGD was experienced as difficult both physically and mentally for Mrs B. This stimulation period of 5 weeks was also difficult for Mr B. because he did not know how to cope, he felt left out. The öocyte retrieval was painless. During the period of 4 days necessary to perform the diagnosis, they both became more and more pessimistic. Finally, they were surprised to hear that two unaffected embryos were available for transfer. Two weeks after transfer, Mrs B. knew that she had not become pregnant.

A few weeks later, at a follow-up consultation, Mrs B. was lost and did not know what to do. For Mr B. it was clear that they would come back for a second PGD trial. They decided to reconsider the different options. For Mrs B. this unsuccessful PGD was again undermining her self-esteem. In response to the question whether they envisaged another spontaneous pregnancy with prenatal diagnosis, both partners had a different view. Mrs B. would like to have another spontaneous pregnancy hoping that this time they would be lucky. She mainly wanted to avoid the whole IVF procedure being too complex and this again reflected her difficulties with taking responsibility for her own actions. Mr B. understood his wife's view but he would prefer PGD. He remembered how difficult it had been for his wife to terminate the previously 'affected' pregnancy. Mrs B. avoided thinking and speaking about these things by remaining silent, pretending there was no real problem. A few weeks later Mrs B. called to announce that she was pregnant. She also claimed that she did not intend to become pregnant now. She was very scared again and did not know whether she would or would not have a chorionic villus sampling. She was not sure whether she wanted to know whether the child was affected. She was completely lost, helpless and distressed. She did not eat or sleep well and was not able to work for 2 weeks. She wanted to deny all the HD-related problems in order not to have to take a decision concerning termination of pregnancy and therefore she was inclined not to have prenatal diagnosis. Finally, her general practitioner convinced her to make an appointment for chorionic villus sampling. Mr B. was not involved in Mrs B.'s thought processes and this led to a crisis in their relationship. Life for Mrs B. was almost impossible. She was very distressed because of the fear of making a decision and because of relational problems between her and her husband. At 10 weeks of pregnancy Mr and Mrs B. were seen again in our centre prior to the chorionic villus sampling procedure. Even then it was not clear for Mrs B. what she would do in the case of an affected fetus. Mr B. remained 'logical' and thought that if the fetus turned out to be affected a termination of the pregnancy should follow. Nevertheless, he was willing to accept and respect any decision of Mrs B. Although no final conclusion was reached concerning their action following a bad result they both wanted to proceed with the prenatal test. One week later, chorionic villus sampling result showed that the fetus was unaffected. This good news did not get through immediately as they both were prepared to hear bad news. Nevertheless, after a period of privacy given to them, Mrs B. said that this was really the first positive experience in her life. However, as the pregnancy and baby may not counterbalance all the previous negative experiences, the value of professional support therapy starting immediately was strongly recommended to them. Mr B. encouraged this suggestion very much and for the first time Mrs B. seemed to be willing to think about the idea. In any case, a close follow-up during pregnancy as well as after delivery was offered.

Comment. This case presents a pathological mourning process in a double way. The first traumatic experience of Mrs B. was the diagnosis of her carrier status for HD. She became stuck in her carrier status, probably because of her restricted social network, possibly also as a result of the lack of a mother figure. As a consequence of the emotional abuse of her mother and the negative test result, she had a low self-esteem and felt worthless. The only thing that, in her eyes, could help her, was finding a husband and having healthy children. This reflects her avoidance of taking responsibility and lack of esteem.

The second traumatic experience was the termination of her first pregnancy after prenatal diagnosis. This also was something she couldn't talk about, because of it being 'taboo'. A lot of symptoms of depression were shown, such as sleep disorder, negative mood, negative self-esteem, internal locus of control and minor physical symptoms, as a result of a mourning process she had not completely dealt with. One of the results of such a pathological mourning process is a problem with the attachment to other people. Mrs B. has realistic attachment problems both to her husband (the fear of being left alone) and to the new fetus (the fear of losing this baby again). Mrs B. became stuck in the process, which impeded her development as an individual being responsible for her own actions. We suggested that this couple go into therapy in order to cope with the difficult topics they have experienced in their life.

2.2 Case 2

Intake. Mr and Mrs S. were referred to our centre in August 2000. They were both 37 years old. Mr S. is a carrier of HD. He underwent presymptomatic testing in 1994 in another genetic centre.

History. In 1993, the diagnosis of HD was made in retrospect in the maternal grandfather of Mr S. His 56-year-old mother was still without symptoms at that time. She refused presymptomatic DNA testing. So the theoretical risk for Mr S. of being a gene carrier was 25%. Despite the fact that Mr S. knew that he had an increased risk, the result that he indeed carried the HD gene came relatively unexpectedly.

Shortly after receiving the unfavourable DNA test result, the couple decided to try to conceive. They had known each other for many years and considered their relationship stable. In the coming years Mrs S. did not get pregnant, probably owing to her disturbed menstrual cycle. Moreover, they experienced serious personal problems. They had just started their own company in gardening tools and were both very busy. Their financial situation was not very good. Nerves were increasingly stretched and therefore they decided to postpone a pregnancy, to take more time to recover from the unfavourable test result and to discuss their future plans, especially concerning family planning, more thoroughly.

A few years later, their situation stabilized and their wish to have children became more urgent. From the beginning, it was clear for both partners that they wanted to have children of their own. Artificial donor insemination and adoption were discussed as possibilities, but were immediately rejected by both. Asked for their motivation for parenthood they answered that their lives would not be complete without children. They considered parenthood to be essential for the further development of their own personalities. Mr S. expressed that in his opinion the social status of couples with children differed significantly from the situation of childless couples. Furthermore, they were convinced that they wanted to avoid HD in their offspring. 'We do not want our children to experience the problems that we are experiencing now.' They both felt a great sense of responsibility towards their future children, and expected they would feel seriously guilty if they would get children without having taken precautionary measures against the transmission of HD. Asked for their future prospective they hope and expect that they raise their children together. Mr S.'s mother is now 62 years old and has HD in its first stage, she is still living independently. His affected grandfather died in his 80s. If Mr S. becomes symptomatic, Mrs S. will take care of both the children and her husband. She describes herself as a strong and independent woman.

In 1999, Mrs S. was pregnant spontaneously for the first time; this pregnancy ended in an early miscarriage. In the beginning of 2000, she was pregnant again. Surprisingly, it was a twin pregnancy and they were convinced that at least one of the twins would be unaffected. Chorionic villus sampling was performed at a gestational age of 11 weeks. Unfortunately, both male fetuses were predicted to be affected with HD and Mr and Mrs S. were very disappointed. The pregnancy was terminated, which was experienced as a heavy burden for both. However, they were convinced that they had truly loved their aborted twins and that they had decided the best they could do for them.

Time went on and in August 2000 they visited our outpatient clinic to again discuss the possibilities of having offspring unaffected by HD and especially the prospects for PGD. They had no principal objection to prenatal diagnosis.

Their main reason for seeking our help was that they felt that they had limited time to have offspring. Mrs S. was 37 years old and they were unaware of how long Mr S. would stay without symptoms. In fact, they asked for PGD because they expected that they would reach their ultimate goal, a healthy child, more quickly and possibly in a more elegant way by means of PGD than by achieving a spontaneous pregnancy followed by prenatal diagnosis. They estimate the burden of an IVF treatment to be equal to prenatal diagnosis with eventual termination of pregnancy. The ultimate decision to undergo IVF with PGD was taken by Mrs S., but Mr S. fully supported her decision. Their intention to undergo PGD was also discussed with their respective parents, siblings and some good friends. They did not want to keep their plans secret and hoped to get some help with this difficult decision. However, they experienced little support from their environment. Their relatives and friends did not understand their situation and regarded IVF/PGD as a 'simple' treatment with 'guaranteed' results. After intensive discussion with their gynaecologist and their clinical geneticist on the advantages and disadvantages, the success rate and the reliability of PGD, they have now decided definitely for PGD and will undergo their first treatment in due course.

2.3 Case 3

Mr and Mrs J. got in touch with us in September 1998. Mr J. was 46 years old at that time and had already had clinical signs and symptoms of HD for some time. In 1996, the clinical diagnosis of HD was made and gene carriership was confirmed by DNA analysis. His father and paternal grandfather also suffered from HD. Shortly after he had received the unfavourable test result he lost his job. Previous personal history further revealed that he was divorced in 1995. He had no children by his first wife. He has a younger girlfriend, and they want to have children. When the couple first contacted our department in 1998, PGD was refused. We had just started PGD and had decided that in this 'pilot' stage we would not treat symptomatic patients; we needed more time to discuss this matter. The couple was seriously disappointed, but continued to regard PGD as the best option in their situation. Mr J. felt a serious objection to prenatal diagnosis and eventual termination of pregnancy. Mrs J. supported her partner in this respect. They both had a positive attitude towards HD, they looked to their future together with confidence and they were convinced that they could give a future child all necessary care. Mr and Mrs J. persisted in their wish to undergo PGD, and have recently reapplied for PGD. We discussed this case repeatedly in our PGD working group and with colleagues, but opinions about whether to go ahead with PGD still differ, and a definitive decision has not yet been taken.

3. Conclusion

It is clear from the previous histories that the decision to undergo PGD is very personal. Couples may have different reasons for choosing PGD, such as an objection to prenatal testing, recurrent prenatal testing with abnormal results and subsequent selective abortion, combined genetic and fertility problems, or presumed 'time saving', as in case 2.

In our experience, most couples take their time to discuss matters seriously, weigh the pros and cons of the different options and are very well able to make a final decision. It is presumably more difficult for future parents to decide to undergo prenatal diagnosis eventually followed by selective abortion, for a late-onset disorder, such as HD, than for early-onset or lethal disorders. Most future parents are fully aware that they prevent the birth of a child who presumably has more than 35–40 healthy years to live, a child that is 'as healthy as the at-risk parent at that moment'. The termination of pregnancy can be felt as a 'denial' of the value of their own lives. In this situation, PGD is possibly a more acceptable alternative, as in PGD selection takes place 'before life'.

Such a difficult situation as in case 1 is unusual among PGD couples, most of our patients do not present a pathological mourning, they are in a stable relationship and are largely supported by family and friends. The second couple has a realistic view on PGD, their limited time to achieve a pregnancy (due to maternal age and the limited 'healthy' time of Mr S.) is one of the main reasons for wishing to undergo PGD. Case 3 raises the question whether or not to offer PGD to symptomatic patients or their spouses. Possible arguments in favour of allowing PGD are that future parents have the right to choose in freedom about their reproductive options. Huntington's disease is a regular indication for prenatal diagnosis, so why not offer PGD, which is even less invasive. Moreover, at-risk persons who apply for PGD are not regularly screened for symptoms of HD, so how can we explain that we refuse couples where we know more or less by chance that one of the partners is symptomatic. However, a possible argument against PGD in these symptomatic patients is that in reproductive medicine we feel a certain responsibility towards the future children. The fact that one of the parents will die at a young age is often used as an argument against artificial reproduction, but in the current situation the future child will also possibly be brought up in difficult circumstances. Our preliminary point of view regarding PGD for symptomatic persons is that it is too early for a general statement. For the time being, it seems most wise to take the decision to accept or reject these couples on an individual basis, after extensive counselling.

Acknowledgements

The authors wish to thank Dr Lize Leunens and Mrs L. Tierney for their contribution and skillful comments.

References

Braude, P.R., de Wert, G.M.W.R., Evers-Kieboom, G., Pettigrew R.A. and Geraedts, J.P.M. (1998) Non-disclosure preimplantation genetic diagnosis for Huntington's disease: practical and ethical dilemmas. *Prenatal Diagn.* 18: 1422–1426.

Maat-Kieviet, A., Vegter-van der Vlis, M., Zoeteweij, M., Losekoot, M., van Haeringen, A. Kanhai, H. and Roos, R. (1999) Experience in prenatal testing for Huntington's disease in the Netherlands: procedures, results and guidelines (1987–1997). *Prenatal Diagn.* **19:** 450–457.

Maat-Kieviet, A., Vegter-van der Vlis, M., Zoeteweij, M., Losekoot, M., van Haeringen, A. and Roos, R. (2000) Paradox of a better test for Huntington's disease. *J. Neurol. Neurosurg. Psychiat.* **69:** 579–583.

Sermon, K., Goossens, V., Seneca, S., Lissens, A., De Vos, A., Vandervorst, M., Van Steirteghem, A. and Liebaers, I. (1998) Preimplantation diagnosis for Huntington's disease: clinical application and analysis of the Huntington's disease expansion in affected embryos. *Prenatal Diagn.* **18:** 1427–1436.

9

Ethical aspects of prenatal testing and preimplantation genetic diagnosis for late-onset neurogenetic disease: the case of Huntington's disease

Guido de Wert

1. Introduction

Prenatal testing and selective abortion are topical issues in biomedical ethics and societal debate. Prenatal diagnosis for late (adult)-onset disorders is especially controversial. This chapter concentrates on the ethics of prenatal testing for Huntington disease (HD), which is often seen as the paradigm case of adult-onset, dominant, neurogenetic disorders. The next section presents some general reflections on the task of the counsellor, more in particular on the principle of non-directiveness (section 2). The following sections focus on the main ethical aspects of the various methods of prenatal testing and preimplantation genetic diagnosis (PGD) for HD (sections 3 and 4). The fifth section sketches some implications for and dilemmas regarding prenatal testing for other late-onset neurogenetic diseases, and the final section briefly comments on the ethical aspects of (still very speculative) fetal neural tissue transplantation *in utero*, aiming at the primary prevention of HD.

Prenatal Testing for Late-Onset Neurogenetic Diseases, edited by G. Evers-Kiebooms, M. W. Zoeteweij and P. S. Harper

2. Reproductive autonomy and the ideal of non-directive counselling

In modern Western culture there is a (strong) consensus that the reproductive freedom of prospective parents should be respected and protected. This so-called 'liberty right' also comes to prospective parents at high risk of conceiving an affected child. At the same time, there is an ongoing ethical debate about the meaning and implications of 'responsible parenthood': should prospective parents at high risk, from a moral (*not legal*) point of view, avoid the birth of an affected child? More specifically: should parents at risk avoid the transmission of the HD mutation? There is little support for the view that prospective parents should take into account primarily societal, in particular economic, interests – a view which would entail an economic rationalization of the notion 'responsible parenthood'. The ethical debate concentrates on the question whether prospective parents at high risk of having a child with (or carrying) a serious disorder should avoid harm/suffering to the future child (Brock, 1995).

Assessing the ethical dimensions of reproductive choices is a complex, difficult and controversial task (Arras, 1990). We must first identify the crucial elements of any assessment and then attempt to weigh and balance them against one another. Important elements include: (i) the magnitude of the possible harm, (ii) the probability of the harm actually occurring, and (iii) the ability and willingness of parents to assume their proper responsibility for the future child. Although the list of relevant elements is uncontroversial, the task of weighing is complicated by the absence of clearly defined standards within each rubric (e.g. 'what risks for progeny are acceptable?') and by the absence of a well-established rule for ranking the importance of each element. In view of this, it is no surprise that reasonable people will often evaluate specific reproductive choices in a different way.

What about the moral responsibility/task of the doctor involved in counselling clients at risk for HD? The professional standard of clinical geneticists/genetic counsellors stresses the importance of non-directiveness to promote the client's reproductive autonomy (Andrews *et al.*, 1994; British Medical Association, 1998). Unfortunately, various definitions of '(non-)directiveness' can be found in the literature. Kessler (1992), for example, defines directiveness as 'persuasive communication in which there is deliberate attempt – through deception, threat or coercion – to undermine the individual's autonomy and compromise his or her ability to make an autonomous decision.' This definition is far too narrow. According to the dominant view, the counsellor has a professional duty to create an atmosphere in which clients can make choices based on their own beliefs, values and preferences. Counsellors should provide unconditional support, whatever the clients decide. Clients may decide to have genetic testing or not, they may decide how to use the information and/or test results they receive as they see best. The counsellor should not give his personal view, at least not unsolicited. To give unsolicited advice, to give one's personal opinion, is, according to Ethics Committee of the Royal Dutch Society of Physicians, unwarranted and unwise, for various reasons.

(i) Recommending any particular course of action undermines the autonomy of the individual client (even though unsolicited advice is not necessarily a usurpation of the client's decision-making authority).

(ii) There is no golden standard for 'genetic responsibility' or 'responsible parenthood'. Reasonable people may regularly disagree about acceptable 'harm–probability' ratios.

(iii) Directive counselling entails a revival of the classical role of the eugenically motivated 'gatekeeper' – which might increase the resistance to genetic counselling (Royal Dutch Society of Physicians, 1997).

In the next sections, where specific types of prenatal and preimplantation testing for HD are discussed, I scrutinize the presumed duty of the counsellor/doctor 'to give unconditional support whatever the client decides'. Here, I briefly indicate three views which qualify the ideal of non-directive (reproductive) counselling.

First, the so-called '(moral) education' model of non-directive counselling, developed by the American philosopher John Arras (1990). This model is based upon a distinction between autonomy as the client's right of final decision-making, which it respects, and unfettered autonomy in the process of deciding, which it rejects. Although counsellors would not tell/advise the client what to do, and although they would respect the final decision of the client, they would attempt to confront the client with the moral dilemmas the client actually faces. So this model allows, or even requires, the counsellor to direct the client through a value-based scrutiny of the available options, playing an active role in expanding the client's awareness of the evaluative issues posed.

This model does not necessarily undermine reproductive autonomy. It may even increase reproductive autonomy by contributing to genuinely informed decision-making. Nevertheless, this model raises some questions that need further scrutiny (De Wert, 1999b). What is it, for instance, about the risk that this education model entails *de facto* 'covert prescripts'? Clearly, there is a fine line between moral education, on the one hand, and recommending a specific decision on the other hand. Furthermore, because of practical constraints, the counsellor will not (always) be able to address *all* the ethical aspects and issues involved. If the counsellor makes a selection of the normative questions to be addressed, which criteria will/should he use for this selection? Isn't there a serious risk that the moral dimension of the diverse options will be narrowed because of the particular moral beliefs of the individual counsellor? Furthermore, it is important to realize that *discussion* on the part of the counsellor has the potential to function as *coercion* in the life of the client (Yarborough *et al.*, 1989). After all, the psychological dynamics of the clinical setting can undermine the equality between client and counsellor. Another set of questions concerns the responsibility of the counsellor to respect the final decision of the client. More in particular, Arras' moral education model, like the 'classical' non-directive approach, raises questions regarding the presumed responsibility of the counsellor to give *unconditional* support – *whatever the client decides/requests*.

The second example of a more differentiated way of thinking about (non-)directiveness can be found in the recent report of the Ethics Committee of the Royal Dutch Society of Physicians (Royal Dutch Society of Physicians, 1997). While the committee stresses the importance of the ideal of non-directiveness, at the same time it acknowledges that there might be exceptions to this ideal – 'never, say never'. In 'extreme risk' situations the doctor may give his unsolicited opinion/advice, i.e. situations in which there is a high risk of devastating harm for the future child. In view of the objections to and risks of directiveness, the Commission stresses that directiveness can be allowed only in exceptional cases and on *some conditions*:

(i)   the counsellor should stress that he gives his personal opinion;
(ii) he should try to influence the client only by rational (non-coercive) persuasion;
(iii) he should discuss these exceptional cases in the team, or ask a second opinion (in order to avoid altogether subjective recommendations).

The Commission does, unfortunately, not give specific examples to illustrate its view.

And third, one may wonder whether the principle of non-directiveness is fully applicable to the practice of *medically assisted* reproduction. After all, the doctors involved have the responsibility to take into account the interests of the future child who will be conceived as a consequence of their own professional assistance (British Medical Association, 1998; De Wert, 1998b, Pennings, 1999). In the UK, this is even a legal requirement under terms of the Human Fertilization and Embryology Act (1990). This means that respecting the autonomy of parents-to-be applying for medically assisted reproduction is an important *prima facie* principle, but not an absolute one. The right to procreate (a so-called 'liberty right') cannot be claimed as a foundation of an absolute right to medical assistance in procreation. The professional responsibility of the doctor precludes a strict adherence to the 'strong' version of the principle of non-directiveness, i.e. the (presumed) responsibility to give unconditional support to clients, whatever they decide (see section 4.2).

3. Prenatal testing for Huntington's disease

3.1 Some preliminary considerations

Prenatal diagnosis is controversial, mainly because of its link with abortion. Objections come from different perspectives, including, first, the so-called 'fetalist' perspective, which focuses on the moral status of the fetus, and second, the disability rights perspective. Let me very briefly review these objections/perspectives.

The status of the fetus. There is considerable difference of opinion with regard to the ontological and moral status of the fetus. At one end of the spectrum are the so-called 'conceptionalist' view (arguing that 'human personal life starts at fertilization') and the 'strong' version of the potentiality-argument: 'because the potential of the fetus to develop into a person, the fetus ought to be respected and protected as a person'. According to these views, (selective) termination of pregnancy cannot be justified (although some authors, assuming for the sake of debate that the fetus is a person, argue that termination could be acceptable/warranted in some cases, e.g. when the women is not responsible for being pregnant) (Thomson, 1971). At the other end of the spectrum we find the view that the fetus as a 'non-person' ought not to be attributed any moral status at all. As a consequence, (selective) abortion is perceived as a morally neutral, 'self-regarding', act. In between these extremes are different other positions. Here a kind of 'overlapping consensus' exists: the fetus deserves a real, but relative protection. The most important arguments are the moderate version of the potentiality-argument and the argument concerning the symbolic value of the fetus. There is a 'strong' consensus that abortion can be morally justified, if there are 'good reasons'. According to the dominant ethical view, preventing the birth of a seriously handicapped child may be one of these 'good' reasons. It is important to realize, however, that some commentators argue that *selective* abortions are ethically more problematic than traditional ('*non*-selective') abortions (i.e. termination of unwanted pregnancies). The 'disability rights' critique, for instance, argues that the practice of selective abortion is at odds with the interests of handicapped people.

Implications for handicapped people.   Prenatal testing and, more in particular, selective abortion are being criticized from the disability rights perspective as they conflict (according to this charge) with the rights and interests of disabled people. Several distinct objections can be discerned in this critique (Buchanan *et al.*, 2000). I mention just a few of these.

According to some critics, selective abortion discriminates against the handicapped, and entails a denial of their equal worth and even their very right to exist. We question the presumed logic of this objection. After all, it is not only *handicapped* fetuses that are aborted. Thousands of healthy fetuses are also aborted, for example, if they constitute a threat to the health or welfare of the mother. But this does not lead to the view that any adult that is a threat to someone's health or welfare is less worthy of respect. The important boundary here is that between fetuses and adults, not between handicapped and healthy (Chadwick, 1987).

Another objection is the '*loss of support*' argument, i.e. the charge that as the use of genetic technologies reduces the number of persons suffering from genetic disorders, public support for the disabled will dwindle. We think it is unwarranted to construe a conflict between, on the one hand, the needs and rights of prospective parents who want to decrease their risk of having a handicapped child and, on the other hand, the interests of disabled people. There, clearly, is a social obligation to maintain, and even to improve, support for disabled people, but it is a *non sequitur* to argue that this generates a claim on the part of those individuals that society must ensure that their numbers do not decrease.

I, therefore, conclude that neither the fetalist perspective nor the disability rights perspective generates valid categorical moral objections to prenatal diagnosis and selective abortion.

3.2 Various types of prenatal testing

Let us now focus on the ethics of prenatal diagnosis for HD: what are the moral aspects? Can prenatal diagnosis for HD be morally justified, and if yes, on what conditions? Below, I consecutively scrutinize the various types of prenatal testing for HD.

Direct ('full') prenatal testing.   The ethics of direct prenatal testing for HD concentrates on three issues. First, is it morally justifiable to abort a fetus carrying the HD mutation? Second, what about prenatal testing for HD 'just for reassurance'? And third, can direct mutation analysis of the fetus without prior knowledge of the genetic status of the at-risk parent be considered as 'good clinical practice'?

Abortion because of Huntington's disease – a quest for perfect babies?
There seems to be a strong consensus concerning the acceptability of prenatal diagnosis and selective abortion for two categories of diseases: first, lethal childhood disorders, such as Duchenne muscular dystrophy, Lesch Nyhan syndrome and Tay Sachs disease, and second, severely handicapping *non*-lethal conditions which manifest themselves *early* in life (e.g. spina bifida, Down's syndrome). The great majority of current applications of prenatal diagnosis belongs to these categories.

Aborting a fetus carrying an adult-onset disorder is especially controversial, and appears even to be prohibited in some countries (see Chapter 6). Even if an abortion in this case is/would be legally acceptable, some people argue that it is ethically unjustified. Huntington's disease is the paradigm case of this category – even though only a small minority of people at risk for HD opt for prenatal testing. Aborting a fetus carrying the HD mutation has been most explicitly criticized by the American philosopher Post (1991). The child, so Post argues, will have 'many decades of good and unimpaired living. Moreover, the parents of the child are not immediately or even directly affected in the way they would be were the disease of early onset'. Post's reservations about prenatal testing for HD are based on two 'humanistic' considerations: first, our desire not to bring suffering into the world must be tempered by the recognition that suffering is a part of life, and escapes human prevention to a large degree. Technology may prevent our coming to grips with the basic existential reality of contingency from which we never fully escape. Second, we should acknowledge the moral ambiguity of the quest for 'perfect' babies ('perfectionism'), and resist 'the tyranny of the normal'. People who are different and 'imperfect' teach us about the meaning of equality and commitment. We must, according to Post, be highly circumspect about declaring too imperfect those persons who must endure somewhat earlier in life the very sorts of frailties that eventually assault each one of us.

Do these considerations undermine the morality of prenatal testing for HD (aimed at aborting a predisposed fetus) (De Wert, 1990, 1998c, 1999b)? Of course, it would be naïve and a misguided effort to fight against all contingencies of human life. The question is, however, whether carriers of HD, who have a high (50%) risk of transmitting the mutation to their children, have the moral right to prevent this by making use of prenatal diagnosis and selective abortion. In view of the fact that HD is a severe disease, and that the penetrance of the mutation is complete, one may reasonably answer: 'yes, they do'. It is insensitive, if not an insult, to (dis)qualify the avoidance of the transmission of the HD mutation as symptomatic of 'genetic perfectionism'. Of course, carriers of HD will be healthy during three to four decades. One needs to recognize, however, that the prospect of their eventual fate often imposes an extremely severe burden. The objection that carriers of HD 'endure just somewhat earlier in life' the frailties that eventually assault each one of us, is misplaced. Finally, Post completely ignores the perspective of the healthy relatives. Many of us will be deeply moved by the sight of a widow of a HD patient: 'When my husband died after twenty-five years of illness, I felt like a light had finally come on at the end of the tunnel. Now I watch my daughter and see her movements and the light has extinguished' (Wexler, 1992).

Let us now take a closer look at the two other moral issues regarding prenatal testing for HD, which concern the *conditions* for such testing.

Unconditional access to prenatal diagnosis?   In general, prenatal diagnosis should also be available for women (with a medical indication) who do *not* consider an abortion (Andrews *et al.*, 1994; British Medical Association, 1998; Royal Dutch Society of Physicians, 1997). After all, prospective parents may have various legitimate reasons for requesting information about the condition of the fetus. For many prospective parents prenatal testing will bring reassurance, whereas receiving an unfavourable test result before birth may enable parents to prepare for the birth of a handicapped child. Access to prenatal diagnosis should, therefore, not be restricted to those persons who intend to terminate affected pregnancies. Should this principle of 'unconditional access' also apply to prenatal testing for HD?

It is important to see that there are morally relevant differences between the traditional applications of prenatal diagnosis, on the one hand, and prenatal diagnosis for HD (Bloch and Hayden, 1990; De Wert, 1990). Should a fetus prove to be a carrier and should the pregnancy be completed then there is a risk that the presymptomatic child will be harmed by being confronted with very burdensome information. Furthermore, the child's right *not* to know may be violated. This right is an example of a distinctive category of moral rights: the 'rights in trust' or 'anticipatory autonomy rights' (Feinberg, 1980). These rights resemble autonomy rights of adults, 'except that the child cannot very well exercise his free choice until later when he is more fully formed and capable. When . . . autonomy rights are attributed to children who are clearly not yet capable of exercising them, there names refer to rights that are to be saved for the child until he is an adult but which can be violated "in advance" so to speak, before the child is even in a position to exercise them. The violating conduct guarantees now that when the child is an autonomous adult, certain key options will already be closed to him.'

Theoretically, it is, of course, possible that the parents will *not inform* the child about its genetic status. In practice, however, there is a considerable risk of the child getting informed without having asked for it.

Fortunately, clinical experience shows that when the implications of prenatal testing for HD are explained to parents who do not consider termination of pregnancy to be an option, they usually decide not to pursue prenatal testing (Adam *et al.*, 1993). This finding highlights the importance of in-depth counselling in order to explain the intricacies and complexities of prenatal diagnosis for late-onset disorders.

But what if parents (who do not consider termination to be an option) insist, and urge the counsellor to give access to prenatal testing for HD 'just for reassurance'? Is it allowed/justified (or even imperative) to make an exception to the rule of unconditional access or not? The lack of consensus is clearly illustrated by the conclusions of various commissions. Guideline no. 7.2 of the IHA/WFN Guidelines states: 'The couple requesting antenatal testing must be clearly informed that if they intend to complete the pregnancy if the fetus is a carrier of the gene defect, there is no valid reason for performing the test.' (IHA/WFN, 1994). The Health Council of The Netherlands, however, concludes that there is an insolvable dilemma between the right of the child not to know and the interest of the parents in a test result that may be reassuring (Health Council of The Netherlands, 1989). The Canadian 'Royal Commission on New Reproductive Technologies' (RCNRT) argues that the rule of unconditional access also applies here (RCNRT, 1993). Let us look in detail at the arguments given.

The RCNRT believes 'that testing for late-onset disorders is one instance where an exception can and should be made to the general prohibition on directive counselling. If termination is not a choice that the couple would be willing to make, counsellors should ensure that the potential harms to the child of knowing the PD test results are clearly outlined to the parents. The facts usually act as a strong deterrent to having testing, and, when parents are unwilling to consider termination, counsellors should discourage testing and explain why they are doing so.' (RCNRT, 1993). The RCNRT does believe, however, that the test should be available, after appropriate counselling, to all eligible couples who request it even if they say in advance that they will not terminate an affected pregnancy. In fact (to some degree), this guideline may be a good example of Arras' *moral education model* of non-directive counselling, which requires the counsellor to confront clients with the moral dilemmas they actually face, but at the same time to finally respect their right of final decision making (see section 2). According to the RCNRT, 'requiring a commitment' to terminate is inappropriate for the several reasons:

1. Most parents can be relied on to make sensible judgements in light of their own circumstances. In fact, the available evidence shows that after appropriate counselling, most couples who reject the option of abortion decide not to have pre-symptomatic PD testing. Commissioners believe that, after appropriate counselling, few if any who would not contemplate termination would be likely to want prenatal testing.
2. It is often difficult for people to know what they will do in a given situation as long as it remains hypothetical. (. . .) It is possible that some women and

couples faced with an actual finding that the fetus is affected would opt for termination, even if they previously thought they would not do so.

3. There is no way to enforce a commitment to terminate a pregnancy. If a woman says that she plans to terminate an affected pregnancy, perhaps to gain access to the test, then decides to continue the pregnancy, she cannot be compelled to terminate. Moreover, it would be unacceptable to try to create a legal mechanism that could compel her to undergo abortion.

4. Finally, the number of couples who might decide to have the testing even if they would not abort is extremely small. (. . .) It is therefore important to keep this issue in perspective.' (Royal Commission, 1993)

Are the arguments of the RCNRT convincing? I doubt whether this is the case. Of course, we all know that many prospective parents who do not consider a termination will refrain from prenatal testing for HD, that it is difficult for people to know what they will do in advance, that enforcing termination is abhorrent, and that we should keep the issue in perspective. But isn't the conclusion that, in view of this, the principle of unconditional access should apply here simply a *non sequitur*? Furthermore, one may doubt whether the position of the RCNRT is *coherent*. If prenatal testing for HD violates the rights and interests of the future child, and should (according to the RCNRT itself) be discouraged by the counsellor, why, then, should the counsellor be *(morally) compelled* to perform the test if prospective parents insist?

Clearly, the opposite conclusion, that *conditional* access to this test is morally justified, or even morally imperative, entails an exception to (or qualification of) the 'strong' interpretation of the principle of non-directiveness, which includes the professional's responsibility to give 'unconditional support' to their clients, whatever they decide.

The objection to prenatal testing for HD on the request of prospective parents who do not consider an abortion entails an analogy between presymptomatic testing for HD in children (which most authors/commissions consider to be unacceptable) and prenatal testing. After all, the timing of harm is irrelevant. Some researchers, however, think that presymptomatic testing for HD in young children might be justified. I presume that they might also accept prenatal testing for HD when parents do not consider an abortion. Michie, one of the proponents of 'empiricism', doubts whether the child will be harmed by predictive testing (Michie, 1996): 'This *may* be true, but it may not be: we lack the evidence. There may also be benefits, such as giving more opportunity to prepare psychologically and practically for the future. Until we know what the actual, rather than the possible, effects are, we should avoid basing policy on speculation. (. . .) Since there is no evidence of testing harming children, we cannot say that taking one or another course of action is more protective.' Of course, testing (very) young children removes the individual's future right to make its own decisions about testing as an autonomous adult. But, so Michie argues, 'untested children lose their right to be tested; and adults lose their right to have been tested in childhood.' Michie concludes: 'Caution in the absence of evidence is 'second best'.

Although one should applaud the development of 'evidence based clinical genetics', one should at the same time acknowledge the risks of this empiricism. I tend to conclude that the predictive testing of young children for HD amounts to an experiment with *disproportionate* risks for the well-being of the child (incompetent research subject), in view of the combination of speculative benefits on the one hand and very real risks on the other (De Wert, 1999b).

Direct testing the fetus of a person at risk?   The international guidelines state that 'it is essential that antenatal testing for the HD mutation should only be performed if the parent has already been tested' (IHA/WFN, 1994). (The guidelines add that prenatal exclusion testing may be a possible exception to this guideline. See below) In other words, it is recommended that centres should abstain from direct mutation analysis of the fetus without prior knowledge of the genetic status of the at-risk parent. I assume that this guideline aims at protecting the at-risk person from psychological harms resulting from a 'double positive' test result that simultaneously reveals that the fetus as well as the at-risk person himself carry the mutation.

Should counsellors really (categorically) refuse to give access to direct prenatal mutation analysis for *paternalistic* reasons, i.e. *on the basis of the 'best interest' of the client*? Ethical theory discerns between *'weak'* and *'strong'* paternalism (DeGrazia, 1991). Strong paternalism is the view that it can be right to interfere with a person's substantially autonomous decision for his or her own good. Weak paternalism holds that it can be right to interfere with a person's less-than-substantially autonomous decision-making for his or her own good. Weak paternalism is not really controversial, because it involves no major violation of the principle of respect for autonomy; those whose wishes and preferences are overridden are acting with less than substantial autonomy. The issue of real controversy is strong paternalism. Some consider such paternalism to be justifiable too, on the condition that:

(i) there is substantial evidence that otherwise the client will be in grave danger;
(ii) the overriding of the client's wish offers a reasonable prospect of bringing about a net benefit to him or her;
(iii) such overriding is the least restrictive way to achieve the desired protection of his or her best interests.

Critics consider strong paternalism to be unjustified because it insufficiently respects the clients' well-considered, subjective weighing of benefits and harms, risks and chances, of submitting to the test.

Let us assume that strong paternalism might be justified on the conditions just mentioned. The question, then, becomes whether the current exclusion criterion for access to prenatal mutation testing meets these conditions. With regard to the *first* condition, one may doubt, in view of the current lack of reliable data, whether there is substantial evidence that the applicant at risk would be in grave danger if he or she were to receive the combined bad news that both the fetus and the applicant carry the mutation.

In order to determine whether the IHA/WFN exclusion criterion meets the *second* condition, we should take into account the burdens and cons of the various *alternative* options, including: (i) no test, just carry the pregnancy to term;

(ii) no test, just terminate pregnancy; (iii) 'sequential' testing, i.e. first, presymptomatic testing of the at-risk person; should he/she prove to be a carrier, then prenatal testing can be performed; (iv) prenatal exclusion testing. The first option is difficult to justify, as it deprives prospective parents of the option to prevent the birth of a child that carries the HD mutation. Clearly, this option is not acceptable for some of the couples. The second option is problematic as well, as the majority of the fetuses (75%) would not carry the HD mutation. The third option may not be feasible in all cases, as sequential testing during pregnancy may take too much time. Furthermore, (enforcing) this alternative might well be at odds with the guideline that individuals should choose freely to be presymptomatically tested and not be coerced by, among others, physicians (IHA/WFN, 1994). It is also important to realize that the risk of obtaining a 'positive' result for the at-risk parent is substantially greater than in case of direct prenatal mutation analysis (namely 50% instead of 25%). Finally, we may question the validity of the consent in prenatal testing of an individual who just received the news that he carries the HD mutation. The fourth option is problematic too, as it entails the risk of aborting a fetus that does not carry the mutation (see below).

I come to the following conclusions:

(i)   although prenatal mutation testing without prior knowledge of the at-risk parent's genetic status is not ideal, the *alternative* options carry their own psychological risks and ethical problems, and do not necessarily bring about a 'net benefit' for clients;
(ii) in individual cases, direct prenatal mutation testing might justifiably be considered as an option for at-risk individuals; and
(iii) the IHA/WFN guideline is too restrictive and should be reconsidered (Maat-Kievit *et al.*, 1999).

Obviously, the precise conditions to be imposed need further debate. In any case, pre- and post-test counselling should be available, and follow-up studies to gather data about this type of testing should be performed.

Prenatal exclusion testing.   When it was introduced, prenatal exclusion testing had two advantages (Harper and Sarfarazi, 1985). It was the first realistic method of avoiding transmission of the disease for couples for whom an informative predictive test was unavailable owing to an incomplete family tree. This, however, became irrelevant once direct mutation analysis became available. The second advantage of prenatal exclusion testing was, and sometimes still is, that it offers the chance to ensure that children are free of HD, at the same time protecting individuals at risk from learning potentially traumatic information about their own carrier status.

What about the ethics of this procedure? Should this procedure, as some commentators argue, be rejected on moral grounds? Various perspectives should be discerned:

First, from a *fetalist* perspective it is objected that the traditional justification of selective abortion is being stretched in this situation. If one knowingly refrains from differentiating between fetuses which carry the HD mutation and fetuses which do not carry the mutation, abortion no longer is a *last resort* to prevent the birth of a child with a handicap or defect. The question arises whether aborting a fetus at 50% risk instead of trying to preserve the fetus without the HD mutation is not too high a price for protecting the at-risk person's right not to know. The answer depends on one's view on the moral status of the fetus. Those convinced of a very high moral status of the fetus may regard this practice as an example of trivializing abortion, whereas those who think differently most likely will consider this practice to be justifiable (De Wert, 1993).

Second, exclusion testing has been questioned for *paternalistic* reasons (i.e. in view of the best interests of the at-risk parent). A first consideration concerns the burdens of terminating a wanted pregnancy when the fetus might be perfectly normal: 'Just imagine – you're pregnant or you've fathered a baby, you're attached emotionally, your fantasies are engaged, and now you're confronted with the choice of aborting a baby who might be perfectly normal. How easy will it be for you to become pregnant again? . . . What if it happens again?' (Wexler, 1992). Furthermore, if the test reveals that the fetus is at 50% risk and the pregnancy is carried to term, the person at-risk will be confronted with two burdening messages at the same time when he later develops symptoms of HD, namely that both he himself as well as the child carry the mutation and will be affected. And finally, parents may suffer from regret reactions if they abort a fetus at 50% risk and are eventually found not to be carriers – the abortion had been unnecessary (Evers-Kiebooms and Decruyenaere, 1998; Maat-Kievit *et al.*, 1999).

In order to answer the question whether a moral dismissal of prenatal exclusion testing on paternalistic grounds is justified, or even morally required, it is, assuming that strong paternalism can be justified in some situations, important to check whether this dismissal meets the conditions for justified paternalism mentioned before. First, there seems to be no substantial evidence that prenatal exclusion testing imposes serious risk of harm on prospective parents who have been counselled adequately about the implications of this type of testing. What about the second condition ('the overriding of the applicant's wish offers a reasonable prospect of bringing about a net benefit to him')? It is, again, important to realize that the *alternative* options (namely: no testing at all, just carry the pregnancy to term; termination of pregnancy; sequential testing, i.e. first presymptomatic testing of the at-risk person, followed by prenatal testing if he proves to be a carrier) all carry their own psychological risks and ethical problems, do not necessarily bring about a 'net benefit' to clients, and will be unacceptable (or less acceptable) for at least some couples. The paternalistic criticism of prenatal exclusion testing is, therefore, not convincing.

Third, the perspective of the (future) child. It has been reported (as far as I can see: in one study) that when at-risk clients opt for prenatal exclusion testing, late reversal of a previous intention to terminate pregnancy occurs in a *relatively large* number of cases (Tolmie *et al.*, 1995). In these cases, the child's right not to know may be violated. After all, when the parent develops the disease, the child will definitely become affected too (Bloch and Hayden, 1990; De Wert, 1990a). *If* this finding would be confirmed in other studies, the *higher* risk for (the 'informational privacy' of) future children would be a serious complication of prenatal exclusion testing. (Whether this would constitute an overriding moral objection to prenatal exclusion testing remains, however, to be seen.) Apparently, however, Tolmie *et al.*'s finding is *not* confirmed (see Chapter 3).

I conclude that, from a moral point of view, prenatal exclusion testing might still be a justifiable option in individual cases (Simpson and Harper, 2001). Adequate pre-test counselling and informed consent are, of course, of paramount importance. Various clinics report that even well-educated clients had considerable difficulty in understanding the principles of exclusion testing (Tolmie *et al.*, 1995). It is, therefore, crucial that the counsellor checks whether the couple correctly/really understands the complexities of this procedure. Furthermore, I argue that the exception to the rule of *unconditional* access to prenatal testing (see above) should also apply here.

'Induction and selective reduction of multifetal pregnancy'?   An alternative strategy for 'avoidance' has been introduced by an Italian team: the so-called 'induction and selective reduction of multiple pregnancy' (Brambati *et al.*, 1994). Like preimplantation genetic diagnosis (PGD, see Section 4), this strategy aims at preventing the birth of an affected child while avoiding a termination of pregnancy. Both strategies have been developed to help fertile as well as infertile couples at high risk of conceiving a handicapped child. The present alternative involves four steps: ovarian stimulation, gamete intra-fallopian transfer (GIFT), CVS and selective fetal reduction. This approach is based on the high rate of multiple pregnancies following ovulation induction and GIFT: the higher the number of conceptuses, the higher the chance that at least one or some of them will be unaffected and a termination can be avoided. The probability of having at least one unaffected fetus in recessive conditions increases from 75% with a singleton pregnancy to more than 99% with quadruplets. In the case of dominant disorders, the respective chances are 50 and 94%. Clearly, the genetic test used in this specific context could be either a *direct* ('*full*') test or an *exclusion* test.

According to the Italian experts, this approach has several advantages in comparison with PGD: it has a higher success rate (in terms of pregnancies and 'take home baby rate'), and it is more cost-effective. It is important, however, to acknowledge the problems and pitfalls of this approach, including the following. First, there is, of course, no guarantee that GIFT will result in a multifetal pregnancy. In case of a singleton pregnancy, there is a high risk that the fetus will be affected, and termination of pregnancy has to be considered. Second, in case of a large multiple pregnancy, it will be difficult, if not impossible, to test all the individual fetuses. Sometimes, it may be necessary to perform a ('non-selective') fetal reduction *before* the CVS (Dumez *et al.*, 1991). Third, the risk of losing the *entire* pregnancy after a reduction can not be ignored. The magnitude of this risk increases with (among others) the number of fetuses. Fourth, after the selective reduction, the woman may still be pregnant of three (or even more) fetuses. Therefore, it will sometimes be necessary to further reduce the pregnancy in order to prevent perinatal mortality and morbidity and serious psychosocial harm to the family. And finally, overzealous ovarian stimulation does have deleterious effects even if multifetal pregnancy reduction can be performed. After the reduction, there is still a 'price to be paid' in an increased risk of prematurity and associated morbidity (Evans *et al.*, 1996).

In view of these problems and pitfalls, the claim that this strategy is a 'reasonable alternative' must be seriously questioned.

4. Preimplantation genetic testing

One can discern various types of preimplantation genetic testing, namely: (direct) preimplantation genetic diagnosis (PGD), preimplantation exclusion testing, and 'non-disclosure' PGD. In this section, I consecutively address the ethics of these different types of preimplantation testing for HD. However, I first address the question whether preimplantation genetic testing can be morally justified *at all*.

4.1 Some preliminary considerations

It is widely accepted that regular prenatal diagnosis and selective abortion can be morally justified as a means to prevent serious suffering for the future child and/or the parents/family. Preimplantation genetic diagnosis can be justified as well: Accepting selective abortion while dismissing a selective transfer would, at least at first sight, be inconsistent. One may even argue that PGD is, from a 'fetalist' perspective, less problematic than regular prenatal testing because the preimplantation embryo has a relatively 'low' moral status. One of the arguments in favour of this position concerns the absence of so-called 'developmental individuation': until the embryonic cells are differentiated and organized to become the primitive streak, embryos may split or fuse – there *is* not yet an individual in any sense of the word, biological, legal or moral. In view of this, the 'pre-individual' preimplantation embryo has a lower symbolic value. One might even argue that the potentiality argument *does not apply* to the preimplantation embryo. Buckle (1990) has discerned two kinds of potentiality, namely the power to *become* and the power to *produce*. 'The power to *become* is the power possessed by an entity to undergo changes which are not changes *to itself*, that is, to undergo growth or, better still, *development*. The power to *become* can thus be called developmental potential. The process of actualizing the potential to *become* preserves some form of individual identity. It is for this reason that the potential *to become* is peculiarly appropriate to arguments which are concerned to establish the importance of respecting capacities of a specific individual. The potential *to produce* differs precisely in this respect – it does not require that any form of identity be preserved.' It is, so Buckle argues, precisely the potential to become which figures in the potentiality argument. Thus, the moral status of the pre-individual preimplantation embryo, which 'only' has the potential to produce, is lower than the status of the postimplantation embryo (the embryo 'proper').

Nevertheless, (the development of) PGD is controversial. Objections, which need to be scrutinized, concern, amongst others:

(i) The experimental use of preimplantation embryos. The introduction and further development of PGD is closely related to preclinical research with human embryos. This research aims at investigating the safety of the various biopsy-strategies and the reliability of the diagnostic techniques. Critics object that this involves an unjustified instrumental use of embryos. The dominant ethical view, however, holds that such research may be morally justified in view of the lower moral status of preimplantation embryos.

(ii) The burdens of *in vitro* fertilization (IVF)/PGD. It is a major advantage of PGD that it can avoid traumatic (repeated) selective abortions. At the same time, PGD carries significant disadvantages. First, PGD presupposes assisted reproductive technologies (ART), more in particular IVF/intracytoplasmic sperm injection (ICSI), which is not the most pleasant way to 'make' babies, carries various sorts of risk for women (ovarian hyperstimulation syndrome, multifetal pregnancies, etc.), and has just a moderate 'take home baby rate', namely 10–20% per cycle. Second, PGD is still experimental: the reliability of the diagnostic tests as well as the safety of the preparatory biopsy (or combination of biopsies) remain to be proven. In view of these risks and disadvantages, paternalistic critics of PGD argue: 'PGD is too burdensome, whereas there are reasonable alternatives, like regular prenatal diagnosis'. These critics, however, ignore that balancing the pros and cons of the respective options is highly subjective. For some couples the so-called 'reasonable alternatives', more in particular prenatal diagnosis and selective abortion, are either *a priori* unacceptable or no longer acceptable (after one or more terminations of pregnancy). Furthermore, for *infertile* couples at high risk of conceiving a handicapped child or a child carrying the mutation for a later onset disease, who opt for IVF/ICSI as an infertility treatment, PGD may be far more attractive than a non-selective transfer.

(iii) The additional loss of embryos. It is sometimes argued that the isolated blastomeres, which will be discarded, are totipotent, and, therefore, have the same moral status as embryos (Gezetz zum Schutz von Embryonen, 1990). The presumed totipotency of individual blastomeres at the 6–10-cell stage is, however, highly unlikely (McLaren, 1997). A second version of this argument concerns the unintended loss of embryos as a consequence of 'biopsy-failure'. According to the experts, however, such embryo-loss rarely happens in experienced hands. Furthermore, in view of (a) the relatively low moral status of preimplantation embryos, and (b) the legitimate interests of prospective parents to avoid (repeated) selective terminations of pregnancy, one may well argue that the possible loss of some additional embryos does not constitute an overriding moral objection to PGD.

(iv) The slippery slope. Some critics question the morality of PGD because this technique might result in the selection of embryos for trivial reasons

(Testart and Sele, 1995). This concern is a good reason to scrutinize the indications for PGD, but is not an overriding objection to PGD as such.

It can be concluded, therefore, that there are no valid categorical objections to PGD. In view of the experimental nature of PGD, its potential risks and disadvantages, I want to stress, however, the prerequisite of adequate counselling and of the informed consent of prospective parents applying for PGD. It is of utmost importance that the couple understands the pros and cons of PGD in comparison with regular prenatal diagnosis.

4.2 Various types of preimplantation genetic testing

(Direct) preimplanatation genetic diagnosis for Huntington's disease. Although there seems to be some interest in PGD among (prospective) parents at risk of having a child carrying HD (see Chapters 7 and 8), PGD for HD is controversial. **Should the indications for preimplanatation genetic diagnosis be more restrictive?** It is sometimes argued that the indications for PGD should be *more restrictive* than the indications accepted for regular prenatal diagnosis. A former Bill in The Netherlands, for instance, stated that PGD should only be allowed for serious/lethal *childhood* disorders. Similarly, the Ethics Committee of the German 'Gesellschaft für Humangenetik', to give a second example, suggested allowing PGD in case of a 'serious childhood disorder or developmental defect' ('schwerwiegende kindliche Erkrankung oder Entwicklungsstörung') (Gesellschaft für Humangenetik, 1996). As a consequence, PGD for HD would clearly not be allowed; (How) can such a restrictive policy be justified?

From an ethical point of view, it would be difficult to *a priori* justify stricter indications for PGD than for regular prenatal diagnosis. After all, a preimplantation embryo does not have a 'higher' moral status than a fetus, accordingly, a selective transfer is not more difficult to justify than a selective abortion. Imposing stricter indications for PGD might, however, be justified on the basis of (more or less) *contingent* considerations. Let me briefly review (some of) these arguments (De Wert, 1998):

(i) 'PGD involves a heavy burden, especially for the woman.' This argument is unjustifiably paternalistic. Furthermore, this argument does not apply to *infertile* couples at high genetic risk, who opt for IVF to treat their infertility (see Section 4.1).

(ii) 'The reliability of the tests is unproven.' I presume that the underlying fear concerns (the small but real) risk of false-negative test results, resulting in an affected pregnancy or even in the birth of an affected child. *Even if* the experimental nature of the test should be regarded (for the moment) as a valid reason to 'set limits', the conclusion that PGD should be performed only for (serious) *early-onset* disorders, is a *non sequitur*. After all, the potential burden(s) imposed by a false negative result may be *less* if the condition has a later onset.

(iii) 'The experimental biopsy carries unknown risks to the health of the child.' Obviously, doctors as well as prospective parents should only take risks if they have a good reason for doing so. But what is a good reason? In any case, this argument has become less convincing as clinical experience to date suggests that the biopsy carries no such risk. A systematic anomaly assessment should provide further data (Simpson and Liebaers, 1996).

It may be concluded that the arguments in favour of more restrictive indications for PGD are either logically incoherent or, in view of the clinical experience, weak. Defects or disorders which are 'serious enough' to qualify for prenatal diagnosis should, at least in principle, also qualify for PGD. The question remains, however, whether PGD for *late-onset* disorders raises any new ethical questions because of potential psychosocial risks of the situation of affected families for the welfare of the child (see below).

Maybe, the real ethical question is not whether the indications for PGD should be *more* restrictive than the indications for regular prenatal diagnosis, but whether the indications for PGD could be somewhat *less* restrictive. After all, many consider preimplantation embryos to have a lower moral status than fetuses (Section 4.1). In view of this, one can imagine that at least some of the critics of prenatal testing for HD would consider PGD of HD to be acceptable from a moral point of view.

Assisted reproduction and the interests of the child   Preimplantation genetic diagnosis presumes, of course, medically assisted reproduction (IVF or ICSI). Doctors involved have a professional responsibility to take into account the interests of the future child who will be conceived as a consequence of their own professional assistance (see Section 2). In view of this responsibility, the principle of non-directiveness cannot be interpreted as an obligation to give *unconditional* access to medically assisted reproduction, irrespective of the potential risks for the welfare of the future child. While most people agree on the fundamental importance of the welfare of the child in the context of medically assisted reproduction, the question remains what evaluation principle, which standard, should guide concrete decisions (evaluations of risks). At least three principles can be discerned (De Wert, 1998b, Pennings, 1999):

(i)   the minimal risk standard/the maximum welfare principle: this implies that one should not knowingly bring a child into the world in less than ideal circumstances. Doctors should refuse to assist in reproduction if there is any risk for the well-being of the prospective child. This standard, *in dubiis abstine*, seems to be too high – in fact it would urge doctors to stop assisting in reproduction altogether;

(ii)   the 'wrongful life' standard/the minimum threshold principle: this view holds that assisted reproduction should be refused only if there is serious risk that the life of the child would be so harmful to him or her that no one would want to live such a life. In these cases to be born is itself to constitute a harm to the child and a violation of his or her right to be born with at least a chance for a minimally decent life. It is obvious that this standard leaves very little room for a psychosocial contraindication for assisted reproduction, based on judgements concerning the suitability for parenthood. If every act of procreation that fulfils this standard is considered to be acceptable, we have to accept some very counter-intuitive decisions;

(iii) the 'high risk of serious harm' standard/the reasonable welfare principle: this is an intermediary principle that avoids the counterintuitive implications of the two other principles. It is, according to this principle, irresponsible and wrong to expose future children to high risks of great suffering. This standard refers not to the perfectly happy child, but to the reasonably happy child. The amount of welfare of the child may be lower than the level that could be expected in ideal circumstances but it may still be optimal given the concrete circumstances and characteristics of the parents. In other words: the welfare of the child might not be as high as it could have been (i.e. had the child had different parents) but it is sufficiently high to be considered a positive gift to the child.

Let us now focus on the case of a (presymptomatic) HD carrier who applies for medically assisted reproduction, whether or not combined with some type of preimplantation testing. Potential risks for the welfare of the future child include *genetic* as well as *psychosocial* risks.

The request of a (presymptomatic) carrier of HD (and even of a person at 50% risk of carrying HD) to get access to assisted reproduction may pose an ethical dilemma for doctors involved (Braude *et al.*, 1998). After all, in view of the fact that a carrier will inevitability develop HD, competence as a parent will be lost steadily with increasing burdens on the other parent (partner). This may have adverse implications for any child born into this relationship. Furthermore, the child may well be confronted with the extreme suffering and death of the affected parent at a relatively young age. Do these psychosocial risks constitute an overriding argument not to assist in the reproduction of prospective parents carrying the HD mutation?

Needless to say that the situation may be burdensome for the child. At the same time, however, it is well-known that many children of HD families are able to cope reasonably well with the situation. Relevant variables include the coping skills of the parent not affected by HD, the quality of the network of the family, the availability of social support, and the age of onset of the disorder in the parent. Clearly, in many cases the child will be an adolescent or even an adult when the parent who carries the mutation becomes symptomatic. In view of this, medically assisted reproduction may well be justified (according to the third, intermediary, standard). Another question which needs further discussion, is whether it would be 'good clinical practice' to offer a neurological examination to an asymptomatic carrier, in order to get information about the progress of the process of neurodegeneration, and if so, on what conditions. Although such examination might be useful for estimating the number of years that the carrier could remain unaffected, and, thus, for quantifying the psychosocial risk for the potential child, the (result of this) examination can be very distressing and confronting for the carrier, as it may result in an early diagnosis of HD.

And what if the prospective father or mother is already *symptomatic*? In this case, psychosocial risks for the future child may be greater, as the child would be confronted with the agony of this progressive disorder 'right from the start'. Should the presence of symptoms of the disorder be used as an exclusion criterion for assisted reproduction? I presume that at least some of the doctors involved will give an affirmative answer. Clearly, doctors cannot be forced to assist in reproduction in these difficult cases. I am, however, not convinced, as yet, that to assist in reproduction would be completely morally unjustified in *all* cases. Further discussion is needed to see whether the variables just mentioned (and maybe other variables) would allow decisions to be made 'case by case'. Questions needing further scrutiny include what experts think about the magnitude of the risks for the welfare of the child, and whether particular risk factors can be identified and used to develop differentiated guidelines. [Another question is, of course, whether a pregnancy may (seriously) worsen the condition of an affected woman. If yes, this might constitute a medical contraindication for medically assisted reproduction.]

In the context of regular prenatal diagnosis, the principle of respect for autonomy is of utmost importance. This means, first, that the doctor should not put pressure on prospective parents at higher genetic risk to opt for prenatal testing. Second, in case of a 'positive' result of prenatal diagnosis, prospective parents should be free to decide whether or not to terminate the pregnancy – the doctor should support them, whatever decision they make. When applied to PGD, this normative principle would, reasoning analogously, imply (i) that doctors should never put pressure on prospective parents to opt for PGD, and (ii) that prospective parents should be free to decide whether to accept (potentially) affected embryos for transfer. Clinical PGD practice, however, reveals that respect for autonomy is not unqualified. What, then, is 'good clinical practice'? In order to clarify the present issue, I first comment on the locus of decision-making concerning PGD, and second on the locus of decision-making concerning the transfer (De Wert, 1998c).

There is consensus that genetic counselling should be available for infertile persons at higher genetic risk who opt for infertility treatment, and that preimplantation genetic testing, if technically possible and available, should be offered. There is, however, some dissent with regard to the *goal* of such testing. The offering of preimplantation genetic testing may have at least two different objectives. First, it enables the couple to informed reproductive decision-making, more particularly to prevent the birth of an affected child. Second, genetic testing enables the doctor to take his *own* responsibility to prevent serious harm to children thus conceived. Sometimes, these goals may conflict.

Clinical experience suggests that couples undergoing ICSI are often not very concerned about conceiving a son who might face infertility in his turn. Most couples at risk of transmitting infertility spontaneously argue that by the time their infant would become an adult, not only ICSI but even more sophisticated treatments will be available to enable him to have offspring. According to Schover *et al.* (1998), couples who faced possible late-onset genetic disorders such as HD or familial cancer syndromes typically used similar patterns of reasoning, anticipating that cures such as gene therapy would be available to prevent their children from suffering.

In 'high-risk situations', some clinics give access to infertility treatment only on the condition that the clients consent to preimplantation testing – in order to eliminate or reduce the risk. In these cases, the offer of preimplantation testing is, in fact, a *'coercive'* offer – an offer patients can hardly refuse in view of the adverse consequences for access to ART. This practice is controversial. Critics hold that a 'coercive offer' clashes with the traditional ethics of reproductive genetic counselling, more particularly with the principle of non-directiveness – the doctor should respect the values and preferences of his clients and give unconditional support, whatever they may choose (Meschede, 1995). This objection is not convincing, because it ignores that doctors offering ART have their *own* responsibility to avoid serious harms to the future children (see Section 2). The real issue, then, is not *whether* it is acceptable to 'coercively' offer preimplantation testing to infertile couples at high genetic risk, who apply for ART, i.e. to give access to those couples only *on the condition* that they opt for preimplantation testing, but *when* this is acceptable, which criteria should be used. In general, the greater the magnitude and probability of predicted harm to the future child, the less morally justifiable it is to medically assist in reproduction. Even if we would agree that medically assisted reproduction is morally unwarranted when there is a 'high risk of serious harm' to the future child (the third standard mentioned before), this principle may invite dissent if applied to individual cases.

In any case, I tend to conclude that when infertile clients at high risk of conceiving a child carrying the HD mutation apply for JVF/JCSJ, doctors may justifiably make access dependent upon the couple's willingness to make use of some type of preimplantation testing.

The second issue to be scrutinized is the decision-making authority when pre-implantation testing has an unfavourable or inconclusive result. At first sight, this may seem to be a 'non-issue'. One may, after all, safely assume that doctors and prospective parents agree that severely defective embryos should not be transferred. It is important, however, to realize that couples may insist that embryos be transferred in case of an *inconclusive* result of PGD – especially when there are *no other*, 'definitely healthy', embryos available for the transfer, and the couple is not willing/able to opt for another IVF/PGD cycle. I presume, this might (in exceptional cases) become an issue in the context of preimplantation *exclusion* testing, where the couple might opt for transferring an embryo at 50% risk if there are no 'definitely unaffected' embryos available (see below). It is sometimes argued that the choice, whether to have the embryo replaced, must lie with the potential mother (Dunstan, 1993). In view of the physicians' *own* professional responsibility to prevent serious harm to the prospective child, however, a (partial) shift with regard to the 'locus of decision-making' seems inevitable. At the same time, this shift raises complex moral questions: what standards should be used in overruling the preferences and autonomy of the couple? How to operate in the context of uncertainty with regard to the prognosis of a potentially affected embryo? When would physicians cross the boundary between a legitimate concern for the well-being of the prospective child, on the one hand, and a dubious 'preventive perfectionism', on the other hand?

In view of the potential dissent with regard to (un)acceptable 'harm/prob-ability ratios', it is imperative that the transfer policy of the IVF clinic be discussed with the couple *in advance* of PGD.

Preimplantation exclusion testing.   Preimplantation exclusion testing might be an alternative to PGD for those individuals who prefer not to know their own genetic status (Braude *et al.*, 1998). Embryos at high risk (50%) would be excluded from transfer notwithstanding that half of these embryos would not carry the mutation. It might be argued that this aspect is not unique/specific, as it is analogous to the use of PGD to detect gender in sex-linked disorders, where half of the embryos selected against may not carry the disorder. However, a notable difference is that in the case of sex selection no alternative diagnostic test may be available, whereas in the case of HD, direct PGD is technically possible.

Like prenatal exclusion testing, preimplantation exclusion testing raises ethical questions. A comparative ethical analysis at first sight suggests that preimplantation exclusion testing may be less problematic. After all, the psy-chosocial risks of this strategy appear to be smaller (the risk of terminating a 'healthy' pregnancy is avoided), whereas the moral status of preimplantation embryos is generally considered to be lower than the moral status of fetuses. The fact that preimplantation exclusion testing may exclude healthy embryos from transfer may therefore not be regarded as an overriding moral objection. A further debate is, however, needed about the question whether it is accept-able to provide *expensive* and potentially *risky* IVF/ICSI-PGD in situations in which there is a 50% chance that the future child is not at risk at all, because the parent does not carry the HD mutation.

'Non-disclosure' preimplantation genetic diagnosis.   The desire of clients to avoid the transmission of HD may conflict with and be completely extin-guished by the possible adverse effects of presymptomatic diagnosis in the at-risk parent. In practice, only a minority (10–20%) of individuals at risk apply for presymptomatic HD testing. As a consequence, so Schulman *et al.* (1996) argue, the potential of antenatal diagnosis to reduce the burden of genetic disease in the population, as well as the tragedy of recurrent cases within a family, is seldom realized. According to these authors, PGD now provides an approach in which antenatal testing can be offered without the adverse effects of presymptomatic diagnosis. Couples at risk could be offered PGD without ever being informed of the specific test results. The couples would be told only that embryos were formed and tested, and that only apparently disease-free embryos were replaced. The parents would specifi-cally not be given any information about the number of eggs obtained, the number of embryos formed, the number in which diagnosis is successful, etc. In other words, no information would be given which might provide a basis for inferring whether any embryos with the HD gene were ever identified. Hence, parents would derive no direct or indirect information about their own genetic risk, while PGD, if performed accurately, could reduce the fetal risk to zero.

Schulman *et al.* (1996) have high expectations of this alternative strategy: 'Perhaps it is not too early to consider the elimination of Huntington disease and other extremely deleterious dominant traits as a goal for the 21st century. This proposal is based on our assumption that many patients at risk for HD would seize the opportunity to prevent transmission of the trait to their children if this could be done without disclosure of their own disease status.'

What about the ethics of non-disclosure PGD (Braude *et al.*, 1998; De Wert, 1998c)? Assuming that PGD for HD can reliably be performed, I restrict myself to some short comments. *First*, Schulman *et al.* stress the public health implications of this approach: 'Perhaps, it is not too early to consider the elimination of HD and other extremely deleterious dominant disorders as a goal for the 21th century.' This eugenic perspective seems to be at odds with the (dominant) ethics of clinical genetics, which, indeed, gives priority to the principle of respect for autonomy and to promoting informed reproductive decision-making (Evers-Kiebooms *et al.*, 1996). Preventing the transmission of gene mutations may be the result of reproductive genetic counselling, it is not its (primary) goal. It is, furthermore, a mistake to think that late-onset disorders such as HD can in principle be eliminated – after all, the phenomenon of spontaneous mutations (resp. dynamic triplet repeats) escapes our control.

Second, non-disclosure PGD presents an alternative for (prenatal or preimplantation) exclusion testing, which likewise prevents the transmission of the HD mutation while at the same time respecting the at-risk person's right not to know his/her genetic status. Obviously, non-disclosure PGD would have a major advantage in comparison with exclusion testing, as it avoids aborting fetuses respectively eliminating embryos which have a 50% chance of not carrying the mutation. And *third*: at the same time, however, non-disclosure testing raises troubling issues. The question is, whether this approach can effectively protect the at-risk parent's preference not to know his/her own genetic status – and, if yes, at what financial, medical, and psychological costs? Let us suppose, for instance, that the first PGD cyclus does not identify any carrier embryo. Depending on the exact number of embryos, the statistical risk of the parent at risk may become close to zero. To tell the client this good news would constitute an indirect-and-unintended breach of *other* at-risk clients' right not to know – after all, they may draw their conclusions if they do not receive this good news. For this reason, I assume that one would withhold the good news. The problem, then, becomes, whether one should offer a second (and a third, fourth, etc.) IVF-PGD treatment, whereas the genetic risk has become almost nil.

Another problem arises, when there are no embryos available for transfer in a given cycle, either because all the embryos are carriers of HD, or for other reasons, like IVF failure. The client at risk might, rightly or wrongly, infer that s/he is a carrier. Should one consider a 'sham transfer'?

Suspending a definite stance with regard to non-disclosure PGD, I would, as yet, suggest: 'Das mag in der Theorie richtig sein, taugt aber nicht für die Praxis' (in theory, it may be a good approach, in practice, however, it is problematic).

5. Prenatal diagnosis and preimplantation genetic diagnosis of other adult-onset diseases

The indications for prenatal testing and PGD are controversial, especially the indications for adult-onset disorders. Some commentators have proposed making an exhaustive, detailed list containing all the acceptable indications. This approach seems to be problematic, for various reasons. First, such a list would need continuous updating, in view of the rapid developments in this field. Furthermore, this approach would insufficiently do justice to the personal circumstances and values of the future parents. Even though the subjective point of view of the future parents is ethically important, respect for autonomy is not unqualified. The question 'Where precisely to draw the line?' is, of course, difficult to answer. I suggest that at least three relevant factors should be *simultaneously* considered (American Medical Association, 1994; De Wert, 1990): the severity of the defect/disorder (determined partly by the availability of treatment and/or preventive measures), the age of onset of the disorder and the penetrance of the genetic defect (the probability that the genotype will affect the phenotype) or the level of risk.

It is evident that there are no easy answers when genetic conditions have a variable expression from mild to serious, a variable likelihood of manifestation, and a variable age of onset. Nevertheless, (to mention the two extremes) prenatal testing for a defect which *(nearly) always* results in a *serious* disorder *in midlife* differs in a morally relevant way from prenatal testing for a defect which *may sometimes* results in a *mild* disorder *late* in life.

Can the ethics of prenatal testing and PGD for HD be used for constructing a model for the ethics of prenatal testing and preimplantation diagnosis for other late onset genetic diseases? I would suggest yes – at least in part. The principles of justice and consistency require us to treat identical or similar cases in the same way. Therefore, guidelines regarding prenatal and preimplantation genetic testing for HD can, and even *should*, guide the evaluation and regulation of prenatal/preimplantation testing for other adult-onset disorders which are similar in relevant aspects: untreatable, lethal, manifesting itself in midlife and autosomal dominant. Relevant examples include some of the other neurodegenerative disorders, such as early-onset Alzheimer's disease, hereditary Pick's disease, and various autosomal dominant types of amyotrophic lateral sclerosis (Rowland and Shneider, 2001; Tibben *et al.*, 1997). However, the guidelines regarding prenatal testing for and PGD of HD do *not necessarily apply* to adult-onset disorders which differ from HD in morally relevant aspects, like disorders which are, at least partly, *treatable and/or preventable, multifactorial,* and/or manifest themselves *later* in life. The ethics of these cases need separate attention, and cannot be simply deduced from the ethics of prenatal testing for and PGD of HD. Needless to say, that it is important to place this debate in the proper perspective: prenatal diagnosis will be even more rarely requested in these cases.

An interesting, though still hypothetical, case would be prenatal testing for the susceptibility for the common, late-onset, version of Alzheimer disease. The APOE genotype is the single most important genetic determinant of susceptibility to late-onset, multifactorial, Alzheimer disease. While most of us would consider prenatal testing for this susceptibility to be rather bizarre, some individuals may disagree and apply for this prenatal test. What should a doctor or genetic counsellor do, faced with such a request?

The American philosopher Bonnie Steinbock argues that the principle of reproductive freedom is of paramount importance: 'Reproductive freedom for women means that women have the right to choose to abort even if they choose for reasons that most people consider trivial or frivolous. No physician should be coerced or pressured into performing abortions, but physicians who do perform abortions do not have the liberty to decide when a termination is justified. Physicians . . . should ultimately respect the woman's right to make this decision and her related right to have information that she deems relevant to the decision' (Steinbock, 1998). Steinbock adds that a quite separate question is whether a specific test should be made 'generally available'. With regard to the case at hand, Steinbock, echoing Arras' moral education model of non-directive counselling, concludes that while the doctor may or even should discuss his hesitations and concerns with the client, ultimately the decision should rest with the client, assuming that s/he is willing to pay for it. I will restrict myself here to a brief comment. Steinbock claims, but does not convincingly argue, that procreative freedom includes the right (apparently: an unqualified right) to have *all* the information prospective parents deem relevant for deciding about abortion. As a consequence, she fails to present a proper balance between procreative autonomy, on the one hand, and professional responsibility, on the other hand. To argue that doctors should ultimately comply even with bizarre requests for prenatal testing, *de facto* makes a mockery of medical ethics. As prenatal susceptibility testing for late-onset Alzheimer disease is unjustified, the doctor should not comply with a request for such testing.

Prenatal testing for adult-onset hereditary cancers, such as hereditary breast and ovarian cancer, might even be more controversial than prenatal testing for HD. (It should be noted that members of affected families have until now shown little interest in prenatal testing for the BRCA mutations involved.) After all, the penetrance of these mutations is incomplete, and preventive interventions may effectively reduce morbidity and mortality in carriers (Lancaster *et al.*, 1996). We should, however, resist premature conclusions with regard to preventing the birth of (female) fetuses predisposed to hereditary breast and ovarian cancer. First, although the penetrance of BRCA mutations is incomplete, the penetrance is still very high (50–85%). In view of this, hereditary breast and ovarian cancer is sometimes classified among the 'monogenic variants of multifactorial disease', i.e. multifactorial disorders (partially) caused by highly penetrant mutations (Health Council of The Netherlands, 1997). And second, relevant questions concern the effectiveness of available preventive and/or therapeutic measures, as well as the burden imposed by the respective medical interventions. Unfortunately, the effectiveness of medical surveillance (mammography) is far from optimal. Though the effectiveness of prophylactic mastectomy appears to be high, longer follow-up studies and study of more carriers are necessary to definitely establish the protective value (and determine the long-term complications) of this procedure (Meijers-Heijboer *et al.*, 2001). Furthermore, prophylactic surgery is irreversible, and may have major implications for women's quality of life. One may, therefore, argue that the fear of a prospective parent with a BRCA gene mutation that his or her future daughters may inherit this mutation is far from unreasonable, and that prevention of the birth of children strongly predisposed to hereditary breast and ovarian cancer is not a trivial concern (De Wert, 1998a).

There seems to be some interest among 'at risk' couples in *PGD* for adult-onset hereditary cancers (Delhanty and Harper, 1997). It is regularly argued that, from a 'fetalist' perspective, preimplantation genetic testing is morally less problematic than regular prenatal testing. Some people might conclude that while *prenatal* testing for late-onset disorders which are partly treatable, or which manifest themselves only 'in old age', is unwarranted, *preimplantation* testing for the respective mutations can be morally justified. Clearly, this view underscores the importance of a systematic comparative ethical analysis of prenatal testing, on the one hand, and preimplantation testing, on the other hand.

6. From prenatal diagnosis to prenatal therapy? New tools, new dilemmas . . .

In the decades to come, fundamental improvements in the ways we approach preventing or delaying neurodegenerative disorders are quite likely. According to William Freed (2000), an expert in the field of neural transplantation research, brain repair strategies in early stages of disease, before major structural damage occurs, in combination with strategies to prevent further degeneration, may have an enormous impact on the outcome of neurodegenerative disorders. One application could be fetal neural tissue transplantation for, amongst others, HD. While ongoing clinical trials include only patients actually suffering from this disease, transplanting fetal neural tissue in a *pre-emptive* manner may, according to Freed, well be a future possibility; if grafts are found to be effective, they could be implanted *prior* to the development of HD, in (asymptomatic) carriers. As it seems probable that striatal transplants would be more effective the earlier they are implanted, the tissue could, so Freed speculates, be implanted shortly after birth – or even *before* birth. In this way, the graft could have the maximum opportunity to become integrated in the host brain.

Scientists may well be overoptimistic regarding future progress in the 'war' against neurodegenerative disorders. Nevertheless, it is important to timely discuss the ethical issues involved in Freed's speculations about fetus-to-fetus transplantation for the pre-emptive treatment of HD. Of course, in theory, this potential future option may represent a welcome alternative for selectively aborting the 'affected' fetus. Fetus-to-fetus transplantation could, if truly beneficial, have major implications for the practice and ethics of prenatal testing for HD. This testing, would, I presume, no longer be controversial. But what about the ethics *'hic et nunc'*? Ethical questions to be addressed regard experimental fetal therapy/surgery in general, 'fetus-to-fetus' transplantation in particular, and the application of these techniques to *late-onset* disorders, like HD.

The ethical framework for fetal therapy is relatively well developed (Fletcher, 1992). The overriding immediate issue concerns the medical risks of experiments *in utero*. The crucial question is: What reasons back up a trial of *fetal* therapy for the disorder in question? The risks involved can only be accepted if they are proportional, which means, amongst others, that post-ponement of medical treatment until *after* birth would probably have adverse consequences for the prognosis for the child. A second immediate moral issue concerns the informed consent. Parents may be very susceptible to investigator bias or optimism. It is of utmost importance that parents under-stand the respective pros and cons, of the various options, including post-ponement of the (experimental) treatment until after birth (Flake and Zanjani, 1997).

The ethics of experimental fetal surgery is further complicated if one would transplant human *fetal* tissue. After all, human fetal tissue transplan-tation is controversial, because it is linked with the practice of elective abor-tion. Nevertheless, there is a 'strong' consensus that human fetal tissue transplantation can be morally justified on strict conditions (De Wert *et al.*, 2002). Most importantly, the decision to terminate pregnancy should be sep-arated from the decision to donate fetal remains for transplantation purposes.

Experimental fetal therapy in general, and fetus-to-fetus transplantation, in particular, so far concern *congenital* defects and *childhood* disorders (Touraine, 1996). It is important to realize that fetal therapy for *late-onset* disorders, like HD, would raise additional questions and concerns. Let me briefly indicate just three of these. First, if one would consider to start experimental *in utero* therapy for a *late-onset* disorder, the risk that the exper-iment will cause ('iatrogenic') *congenital* defects will be especially difficult to justify, as the child would otherwise have been healthy for at least a few decades. Second, for future couples interested in fetus-to-fetus transplanta-tion research, prenatal testing for HD would get a new, completely different, ratio, namely discovering whether their fetus could be included in the clin-ical trial. Clearly, if the preventive and/or therapeutic results of the *in utero* transplantation would prove to be disappointing, the future child could well claim that his right not to know has been violated by the preceding prenatal diagnosis. This psychosocial/moral risk should be included in the calculus of potential benefits and harms. And third, fetal experimental therapy for late-onset disorders could only be justified if its effects would be adequately monitored. This would require long-term, extensive, follow-up studies. These studies would raise all sorts of methodological, practical and moral issues, like: how to guarantee long-term participation in these studies? What if teenagers object to further participation? Is it justified to put moral pres-sure on research subjects?

It remains to be seen, of course, whether Freed's speculations will be mater-ialized in the decades to come. If so, it is of utmost importance to scrutinize any future *in utero* transplantation research protocols, and to critically evaluate the claim that this (extremely) proactive approach has a positive risk-benefit ratio.

Acknowledgements

I would like to express my gratitude to Professor G.Evers-Kiebooms and Professor A.Tibben (Erasmus University Rotterdam, The Netherlands) for their useful comments on the draft of this chapter.

References

Adam, S., Wiggins, S., Whyte, P., et al. (1993) Five years study of prenatal testing for Huntington's disease: demand, attitudes, and psychological assessment. *J. Med. Genet.* **30:** 549–556.

American Medical Association, Council on Ethical and Judicial Affairs (1994) Ethical issues related to prenatal genetic testing. *Arch. Fam. Med.* **3:** 633–642.

Andrews, L.B., Fullarton, J.E., Holtzman, N.A. and Motulsky, A.G., eds (1994) *Assessing Genetic Risks. Implications for Health and Social Policy.* National Academy Press, Washington, DC.

Arras, J.D. (1990) AIDS and reproductive decisions: having children in fear and trembling. *Milbank Q.* **68:** 353–382.

Bloch, M. and Hayden, M.R. (1990) Opinion: predictive testing for Huntington disease in childhood: challenges and implications. *Am. J. Hum. Genet.* **46:** 1–4.

Brambati, B., Formigli, L., Mori, M., et al. (1994) Multiple pregnancy induction and fetal reduction in high genetic risk couples. *Hum. Reprod.* **9:** 746–749.

Braude, P.R., De Wert, G. de, Evers-Kiebooms, G., et al. (1998) Non-disclosure preimplantation genetic diagnosis for Huntington's disease: practical and ethical dilemmas. *Prenatal Diagn.* **18:** 1422–1426.

British Medical Association (1998) *Human Genetics. Choice and Responsibility.* Oxford University Press, Oxford.

Brock, D. (1995) The non-identity problem and genetic harm. *Bioethics* **9:** 269–276.

Buchanan, A., Brock, D.W., Daniels, N. and Wikler, D. (2000) *From Chance to Choice. Genetics and Justice.* Cambridge University Press, Cambridge.

Buckle, S. (1990) Arguing from potential. In: *Embryo Experimentation* (eds P. Singer, H. Kuhse, K. Dawson and P. Kasimba). Cambridge University Press, Cambridge, pp. 90–108.

Chadwick, R. (1987) The perfect baby: introduction. In: *Ethics, Reproduction and Genetic Control* (ed. R. Chadwick). Routledge, London, pp. 93–135.

DeGrazia, D. (1991) The ethical justification for minimal paternalism in the use of the predictive test for Huntington's disease. *J. Clin. Ethics* **2:** 219–228.

Delhanty, J.D.A. and Harper, J. (1997) Genetic diagnosis before implantation. *BMJ* **315:** 828–829.

De Wert, G. (1990) Prenatal diagnosis and selective abortion: some ethical considerations (in Dutch). In: *Ethiek en Recht in de Gezondheidszorg* (eds H. ten Have *et al.*). Deel XVI, pp. 121–153.

De Wert, G. (1992) Predictive testing for Huntington disease and the right not to know. Some ethical reflections. In: *Psychological Aspects of Genetic Counseling* (eds G. Evers-Kiebooms, J.-P. Fryns, J.-J. Cassiman and H. Van den Berghe). Wiley-Liss, New York, pp. 133–138.

De Wert, G. (1998a) Ethics of predictive DNA-testing for hereditary breast and ovarian cancer. *Patient Educ. Counsel.* **35:** 43–52.

De Wert, G. (1998b) The post-menopause: playground for reproductive technology? Some ethical reflections. In: *The Future of Human Reproudction. Ethics, Choice and Regulation* (eds J. Harris and S. Holm). Clarendon Press, Oxford, pp. 221–237.

De Wert, G. (1998c) Ethics of preimplantation genetic diagnosis. In: *Genetics in Human Reproduction* (eds E. Hildt and S. Graumann). Ashgate, Aldershot, pp. 75–96.

De Wert, G. (1999a) Ethics of assisted reproduction: the case of preimplantation genetic diagnosis. In: *Molecular Biology in Reproductive Medicine* (eds B.C.J.M. Fauser, A.J. Rutherford, J. F. Strauss II and A. Van Steirteghem). Parthenon Publishing, New York, pp. 433–448.

De Wert, G. (1999b) Assisted reproductive technologies, genetic testing and ethics (in Dutch). Thela Thesis, Amsterdam.

De Wert, G., Berghmans, R., Boer, G.J., et al. (2002) Ethical guidance on human embryonic and fetal tissue transplantation: a European overview. *Med. Health Care Philos.* **5:** 79–90.

Dumez, Y., et al. (1991) First-trimester prenatal diagnosis in quintuplets: a practical approach using step-by-step embryo reduction. *Prenatal Diagn.* **11:** 737–740.

Dunstan, G. (1993) Ethics of gamete and embryo micromanipulation. In: Gamete and embryo micromanipulation in human reproduction (eds S. Fishel and S. Symonds). Edward Arnold, London, pp. 212–218.

Evans, M.I., Dommergues, M., Wapner, R.J., et al. (1996) International, collaborative experience of 1789 patients having multifetal pregnancy reduction: a plateauing of risks and outcomes. *J. Soc. Gynecol. Invest.* **3:** 23–26.

Evers-Kiebooms, G., Fryns, J.P., Demyttenaere, K., et al. (1996) Predictive and preimplantation genetic testing for Huntington's disease and other late onset dominant disorders: not in conflict but complementary (letter). *Clin. Genet.* **50:** 275–276.

Evers-Kiebooms, G. and Decruyenaere, M. (1998) Predictive testing for Huntington's disease: a challenge for persons at risk and for professionals. *Patient Educ. Counsel.* **35:** 18–26.

Feinberg, J. (1980) The child's right to an open future. In: *Whose Child? Children's Rights, Parental Authority, and State Power* (eds W. Aiken and H. LaFollette). Littlefield, Adams & Co, Totowa, NJ, pp. 124–153.

Flake, A.W. and Zanjani, E.D. (1997) *In utero* hematopoietic stem cell transplantation. A status report. *JAMA* **278:** 932–937.

Fletcher, J.C. (1992) Fetal therapy, ethics and public policies. *Fetal. Diagn. Ther.* **7:** 158–168.

Freed, W.J. (2000) *Neural Transplantation. An Introduction.* MIT Press, Cambridge, MA.

Gesellschaft fuer Humangenetik (1996) Positionspapier. *Medizinische Genetik* **8:** 125–131. Gesetz zum Schutz von Embryonen vom 13. Dezember 1990 (BGBI.I S.2746)

Harper, P.S. and Sarfarazi, M. (1985) Genetic prediction and family structure in Huntington's chorea. *BMJ* 1929–1931.

Health Council of The Netherlands (1989) *Heredity: Science and Society.* Health Council of The Netherlands, The Hague.

Health Council of The Netherlands (1998) *DNA-Diagnostics.* Health Council of The Netherlands, Rijswijk (in Dutch).

Human Fertilisation and Embryology Act (1990)

International Huntington Association, World Federation of Neurology (1994) Guidelines for the molecular genetics predictive test in Huntington's disease. *Neurology* **44:** 1533–1536.

Kessler, S. (1992) Psychological aspects of genetic counseling. VII. Thoughts on directiveness. *J. Genet. Counsel.* **1:** 9–17.

Lancaster, J.M., Wiseman, R.W. and Berchuck, A. (1996) An inevitable dilemma: prenatal testing for mutations in BRCA1 breast-ovarian cancer susceptibility gene. *Obstet. Gynecol.* **87:** 306–309.

Maat-Kievit, A., Vegter-Van der Vlis, M., Zoeteweij, M., et al. (1999) Experience in prenatal testing for Huntington's disease in the Netherlands: Procedures, results and guidelines (1987–1997). *Prenatal Diagn.* **19:** 450–457.

McLaren, A. (1997) A note on 'totipotency'. *Biomedical Ethics. Newsletter of the European Network for Biomedical Ethics* **2** (1): 7.

Meijers-Heijboer, H., Van Geel, B., Van Putten, W., et al. (2001) Breast cancer after prophylactic bilateral mastectomy in women with a *BRCA1* or *BRCA2* mutation. *N. Engl. J. Med.* 345: 159–164.

Meschede, D. (1995) Genetic risk of micromanipulative assisted reproduction. *Hum. Reprod.* **10:** 2880–2886.

Michie, S. (1996) Predictive testing in children: paternalism or empiricism? In: *The Troubled Helix. Social and Psychological Implications of the New Human Genetics* (eds Th. Marteau and M. Richards). Cambridge University Press, Cambridge, pp. 177–183.

Nuffield Council on Bioethics (1998) *Mental Disorders and Genetics: the Ethical Context.* Nuffield Council on Bioethics, London.

Pennings, G. (1999) The welfare of the child. Measuring the welfare of the child: In search of the appropriate evaluation principle. *Hum. Reprod.* **14:** 1146–1150.

Post, S. (1991) Selective abortion and gene therapy: reflections on human limits. *Gene Ther.* **2:** 229–233.

Royal Commission on New Reproductive Technologies (1993) *Proceed with Care. Volume I.* Minister of Government Services, Ottawa.

Royal Dutch Society of Physicians (1997) *Doctors and Genes: The Use of Genetic Knowledge in Clinical Practice.* Royal Dutch Society of Physicians, Utrecht (in Dutch).

Rowland, L.P. and Shneider, N.A. (2001) Amyotrophic lateral sclerosis. *N. Engl. J. Med.* **344:** 1688–1700.

Schover, L.R., Thomas, A.J., Falcone, T., et al. (1998) Attitudes about genetic risk of couples undergoing *in-vitro* fertilization. *Hum. Reprod.* **13:** 862–866.

Schulman, J.D., Black, S.H., Handyside, A. and Nance, W.E. (1996) Preimplantation testing for Huntington disease and certain other dominantly inherited disorders. *Clin. Genet.* **49:** 57–58.

Simpson, S.A. and Harper, P.S. (2001) Prenatal testing for Huntington's disease: experience within the UK 1994–1998. *J. Med. Genet.* **38:** 333–335.

Simpson, J.L. and Liebaers, I. (1996) Assessing congenital anomalies after preimplantation genetic diagnosis. *J. Assist. Reprod. Genet.* **13:** 170–176.

Steinbock, B. (1998) Prenatal genetic testing for Alzheimer's disease. In: *Genetic Testing for Alzheimer Disease. Ethical and Clinical Issues* (eds S.G. Post and P.J. Whitehouse). John Hopkins University Press, Baltimore, MD, pp. 140–151.

Testart, J. and Sele, B. (1995) Towards an efficient medical eugenics; is the desirable always the feasible? *Hum. Reprod.* **10:** 3086–3090.

Thomson, J.J. (1971) A defence of abortion. *Philos. Public Affairs* **1:** 47–66.

Tibben, A., Stevens, M, De Wert, G., et al. (1997) Preparing for presymptomatic DNA testing for early onset Alzheimer's disease/cerebral haemorrhage and hereditary Pick disease. *J. Med. Genet.* **34:** 63–72.

Tolmie, J.L., Davidson, H.R., May, H.M., et al. (1995) The prenatal exclusion test for Huntington's disease: experience in the west of Scotland, 1986–1993. *J. Med. Genet.* **32:** 97–101.

Touraine, J.-L. (1996) *In utero* transplantation of fetal liver stem cells into human fetuses. *J. Hematother.* **5:** 195–199.

Wexler, N. (1992) Clairvoyance and caution. In: *The Code of Codes. Scientific and Social Issues in the Human Genome Project* (eds D. Kevles and L. Hood). Harvard University Press, Cambridge, MA, pp. 211–244.

Yarborough, M., Scott, J.A. and Dixon, L.K. (1989) The role of beneficence in clinical genetics: non-directive counseling reconsidered. *Theoret. Med.* **10:** 139–149.

10

Prenatal testing – dilemmas and problems facing Huntington's families. A lay perspective

Sue Watkin and Kees Varkevisser

1. Introduction

The very nature of the International Huntington Association makes for a wide diversity of opinions. The very nature of human beings means that there is little chance of a consensus. To emphasize the diversity, the International Huntington Association is the umbrella organization for the Huntington's disease lay associations around the world. There are more than 35 members ranging from long-established organizations with salaried staff to fledgling societies with a few families and committed professionals.

Whether or not you take a view on prenatal testing may possibly be dependent on its availability, its relevance, its scale in your order of priorities or your moral values. Where there is poverty, isolation, inadequate support and a lack of basic care just coping with Huntington's disease (HD) is a daily struggle. Close to the borders of the European Union there are the countries of Eastern Europe. There support is minimal. There is not enough money to produce printed leaflets to give the facts to families. Within the borders of the European Union there are countries with no lay associations. It is important to remember that although the issue of prenatal testing is important there is a range of wider issues which impinge heavily on families touched by HD.

The risk of developing an illness suffered by your parents or other close relatives at a later stage in your own life is a huge burden. In the 1980s a survey of

Prenatal Testing for Late-Onset Neurogenetic Diseases, edited by G. Evers-Kiebooms, M. W. Zoeteweij and P. S. Harper

Huntington families in Belgium to ascertain how many would ask for predictive testing, should it become available, showed that many more than half the people at risk were very interested and would seriously consider this option (Evers-Kiebooms *et al.*, 1989). When, in 1983, the gene was located on chromosome 4 and predictive testing, by means of linkage analysis, became a possibility, the number of people who requested this test turned out to be considerably smaller than expected. The same phenomenon was seen in many other countries.

People at risk of HD felt differently when confronted by the reality of the test and the fear that they might be confronted with a bad test result. This fear combined with potential problems within family relationships, worries about the information becoming known within the work place or affecting financial matters, such as insurance, may go some way to explaining the low uptake figure. Figures suggest that more than 80% of those at risk preferred 'not knowing' to 'knowing'. At that time, uncertainty was preferable to certainty and nothing has changed since (Chapters 3, 4, 5 and 13).

2. Views and prenatal testing for Huntington's disease

Like predictive testing in adults, prenatal testing (also by means of linkage analysis) was introduced in the second half of the 1980s. This seemed to offer the opportunity to solve another major problem for families affected by HD, i.e. a way to avoid the risk of passing on the gene to their children. However, even smaller numbers of individuals seemed interested in this test and it is likely that several considerations played a contributory role. In the case of an unfavourable test result there is the anguish of termination of the pregnancy. The decision not to burden their child with inheriting HD is rendered more difficult when faced with the decision to end the life of a planned and wanted child. The existence of a pregnancy and the reality of parenthood make this a painful decision. Furthermore, potential parents were and continue to be discouraged from continuing with a pregnancy in which a test had indicated an unfavourable outcome because such a situation would result in the violation of the child's right not to be tested and sits uneasily with the protocol for testing.

As the disease does not skip a generation detecting the HD gene in the unborn child automatically shows that the 'at-risk' parent (who is asymptomatic and has not have a predictive test to detect whether he or she is a carrier) must have inherited the HD gene too. If this parent has already been tested and knows that they have inherited the gene this does not pose a problem. However, it is a major problem for those at risk who want a 'risk-free' child but do not want to have their own genetic status revealed. Under such circumstances prenatal testing is not a viable option. However, the exclusion test goes some way to meeting the wish of the prospective parents to remain ignorant of their genetic status by using genetic information from a number of family members, i.e. parents and grandparents. It turns a 25% risk for the fetus into a 50% risk or a 0% risk. However, a proportion of fetuses given a 50% risk status are in fact free of the HD gene. Furthermore, a problem might arise should the parents decide against abortion of the child whose risk is 50%. As both parent and child have inherited the same chromosome from the 'ill' grandparent, the child would be known to be a gene carrier should the 'at-risk' parent develop symptoms of the disease. Again, this situation results in the violation of the child's right not to be tested. Both of these tests (full prenatal testing to get full information about the presence or absence of the Huntington gene in the fetus and exclusion testing) are difficult options if you are uncomfortable with termination. The exclusion test with the greater probability of terminating a fetus without the HD gene is even more problematic.

Agonizing over whether to have an 'at-risk' child is an emotional rollercoaster. There is no doubt that prenatal testing may take an awful emotional toll. Many couples who are unlucky and have to resort to one or more terminations are traumatized by such events. Many relationships are permanently damaged by these undertakings.

In terms of people who opt for exclusion testing to avoid the knowledge of their own status there are huge problems. Couples who have had several terminations have expressed relief when the 'at-risk' partner develops the disease. At least they can then justify their actions. Couples where the at-risk partner subsequently undergoes predictive testing with a favourable outcome or does not go on to develop the disease may be consumed with guilt or traumatized by the loss of their HD gene-free children.

The discovery of the HD gene itself, in 1993, altered the testing process and allows for predictive and prenatal testing without the need for the cooperation of wider family members. This direct mutation test also provides almost 100% reliability. Laboratory work has become easier and quicker. Similar to full prenatal testing by DNA linkage, the direct mutation test for prenatal testing purposes does not allow a person to use the 'escape mechanism' of an exclusion test. If the fetus has the HD gene, then the prospective, at-risk parent automatically must be a gene carrier too. Their 50% risk status will have changed to 100%. Under these circumstances there is the potential for a double dose of bad news for those undergoing prenatal testing. It is for this reason that the guidelines for prenatal testing state that it should only be carried out after the 'at risk' parent has been tested. The exclusion test continues to be available for persons at risk who do not want to know whether they are carriers of the Huntington mutation.

3. Views on preimplantation genetic diagnosis

The latest technique to assist couples is the advent of *in vitro* fertilization (IVF) combined with preimplantation genetic diagnosis (PGD). Both tests, direct and exclusion, can be performed with this technique and it appears to be a viable alternative to prenatal testing in early pregnancy. However, the major disadvantage of this is the necessity of burdensome and intrusive IVF procedures with all its risks and the emotional burden in the absence of fertility problems.

Prenatal testing is not available in all European countries. The PGD test is only available in a few centres. In some countries abortion is not a legal option. In the booklet, 'Designer Myths – the Science, Law and Ethics of PGD' by Kay Chung (1999) it states, 'There are only 30 or so centres around the world that offer PGD. The slow development of the service is partly due to the technical complexity of the diagnosis and to the multidisciplinary nature of the service (see also Chapter 7). Its relative scarcity as a service is also the result of legal restrictions placed upon it in some countries. There are three main legal approaches to PGD around the world. The first approach is where PGD is permitted but regulated. Second, it is completely outlawed in some countries. The third approach is to allow PGD to take place free from regulation. This range of positions is also represented in Europe where some countries have adopted a fairly permissive legal position on PGD, whereas others have adopted a tougher stance. In some countries, attitudes towards PGD depend on attitudes to the moral status of the human embryo. Germany, Austria, Switzerland and Norway prohibit any kind of research using human embryos and prohibit PGD for the same reason.

Preimplantation genetic diagnosis represents another choice but obviously with limitations depending on where you live. To date, people with a family history of HD have the choice of predictive testing, prenatal testing, now PGD or the option of choosing none. To emphasize the low uptake rate: the uptake for predictive testing in the UK is 15–18% and in 1999/2000 just 24 prenatal tests were carried out in the UK. It is difficult to gauge the extent of the use of PGD. Of course, for couples thinking of having a family there is the further choice of trusting to luck. For some people the only option is not having a family at all. People who find prenatal testing morally indefensible are inclined to have similar views on PGD. Most of these people believe that life begins with fertilization and therefore find PGD unacceptable. They are also unhappy because PGD involves not only the selection of healthy embryos but also the inevitable discarding of affected embryos. However, others have expressed the view that PGD must be preferable to prenatal testing because they feel that life in a meaningful sense does not begin until much later in a pregnancy. Some people have said that PGD is preferable to prenatal diagnosis because the couple knows at the beginning of pregnancy that their baby does not carry the Huntington mutation. Some people say that PGD must be preferable because to have a termination is such a traumatic event. However, many people are uneasy about the emotional and physical stresses of PGD. Most people are aware of the difficulties of IVF treatment for infertility reasons as such treatment has been available for many years. They are concerned because the procedure is unpleasant, is not without risks and gives no guarantee of a pregnancy. They also know that it is likely to be very expensive.

Here are some opinions on PGD posted on HD websites:

Ann writes, 'It seems that it is easier, less of a crime, to dispose of a human life just because it is only eight to ten cells. I think that throwing away a few cells is wrong if we are talking about a human being but everyone is going to do what they want anyway. People seem to find a way to justify their behaviour if they want something badly enough.'

Jean writes, 'This is a personal decision, one not easily made. It is a matter of choice for the families involved. Their decisions should be respected and not questioned by others who have not been in the same position.'

Many people have posed the question 'Is it fair to have a child knowing that he or she will grow up in a family where a parent has Huntington's disease?' The most common retort is that a couple could choose to have a child anyway – it doesn't need to be through prenatal testing or PGD. But centres offering PGD have a duty to consider the welfare of the child or children. Children's well-being is a major cause for concern. Most of the really difficult work undertaken by lay associations relates to children. The most harrowing situations involve the care of children when a parent is no longer able to cope. People with HD often face not only the loss of their partner, but may also lose their children in custody battles. Children face being young carers, face the bewilderment of seeing a dearly loved parent changing before them, they may worry about bringing their friends home. These children may suffer unintentional neglect, verbal and often physical abuse. But children will face these problems whether the result of PGD, prenatal testing or leaving things to chance. The only difference for the first two groups is the comforting knowledge that HD will not be their fate.

Professionals involved with PGD have said that people undergoing this difficult procedure in order to have a child free of the HD gene are likely to be especially committed to the welfare of their children. Most have the best interests of their children at heart whether HD is part of their lives or not. Huntington's disease disrupts relationships. Families will have difficulties, however good their intentions.

Compared with prenatal testing PGD is expensive. People both inside and outside the Huntington's community wonder how this treatment will be funded. 'Who is this treatment available to – gene positive people, at risk people, symptomatic people, wealthy people?' Most centres will make PGD available to at-risk couples. When eliciting views from people this is a subject which generates a great deal of controversy. Many people believe that no one should go through this unpleasant and invasive procedure when it might not be necessary. They question whether anyone should ask his partner to do this. For both the man and the woman there are a lot of emotional issues surrounding this procedure. For the woman there is a lot of physical discomfort and even risk. The other side of the argument says that if prenatal exclusion testing is ethically and morally acceptable then PGD for the 'at-risk' person must be acceptable as well. However, some people may feel that this is a waste of resources.

With PGD there is the additional problem of multiple births. Some centres have decided that a maximum of two embryos will be implanted. What happens if the couple wants three, perhaps because they think it improves their chances of a successful pregnancy, maybe because they are older and feel that time is passing them by, maybe because they can't afford another attempt. There will then be the practical difficulties of multiple births.

And there is another group of people – the symptomatic. Some centres offering PGD have a neurological assessment of the at-risk or gene-positive person as part of their protocol. Centres have said people will not be excluded on the grounds that they are symptomatic alone. It is possible that they will be discouraged. One has to question the likelihood of PGD being available to them. One might question whether it will be looked upon more or less favourably, depending on whether the symptomatic person is the potential mother or the potential father. If so, perhaps disability discrimination law would be breached. Alternatively the welfare of the child could be invoked.

Then we come to the problem of funding this treatment. Will people's hopes be raised only to be dashed because they can't afford to pay? In the UK prenatal testing is paid for by the NHS. How will PGD be funded? Most health authorities don't pay for IVF treatment – will they pay for PGD? If they do how many attempts will be paid for? It is likely that people in other countries will face this problem too. And what of people who live in countries where this procedure is illegal? Will this be yet another option only available if you can afford it?

Furthermore, in relation to PGD there is another test possibility for at risk family members, namely a non-disclosure test. In this instance, fertilized, HD gene-negative eggs could be transferred without giving any information that might disclose the status of the at-risk parent. In theory, this appears an attractive alternative but there would be many ethical problems: if all the embryos were shown to be HD gene-negative in a series of tests, this might indicate that the 'at-risk' parent was not a gene carrier. Should they then be informed that the procedure might well be unnecessary? If another member of the same family or a friend undergoing PGD was not given similar information they would conclude that they were gene carriers. In another scenario all the embryos could be shown to be HD-positive (which may occasionally happen, especially if the number of eggs is small). Should the doctor consider a sham transferral of embryos? Alternatively, if the parent is told that there are no HD gene-free embryos, the parent will suppose that they have inherited the gene, thus undermining the purpose of pursuing this particular test to maintain one's own at risk status.

4. Pressures to test

How much of an emotional toll do all these procedures take on relationships? All kinds of reasons are cited for the low uptake of prenatal testing but it is possible that the main reason is that people just want to be normal. They just want to have children in the time-honoured way. They want to go along for the 3-month scan and look with wonder at their developing child. So these are the options available to couples. How realistic is it to believe that parents can make their choices unencumbered by outside pressure? Pressures come from many directions and take many forms. Conflict may exist within a couple's own relationship when one person insists on a child free of the risk of HD and perhaps the other person prefers not to know there own status or does not believe in abortion.

Pressure may come from wider family members whose own experiences of living with HD makes them believe that it is morally wrong to take the risk of bearing a child with the HD gene. In a recent HDA Newsletter article in the UK a contributor writes, 'Despite a Catholic upbringing, I think it is wrong to bring into the world a child condemned to develop a devastating, incurable dis-ease if there is any way of ascertaining the presence of the mutant gene before the child is born. I admire anyone who is willing to suffer in person for his or her principles, religious or otherwise. What is not acceptable is to condemn someone else to suffer (in this case one's own children).'

There is the pressure of time when a woman is already pregnant when she is referred to the genetic clinic. Prenatal testing with all its possibilities and consequences takes time to absorb, think about and discuss. Decision-making under pressure is not always the best approach.

Friends, the family doctor or specialists may bring pressure to bear upon a couple considering a pregnancy, dependent on their own perspectives. The prevailing attitudes of society contribute to the pressure. Many people believe that if the technology exists it must be used. Women who have continued with a Down's syndrome pregnancy are made to feel irresponsible. Women who refuse prenatal screening often feel that they need to apologize for their decision.

There is also the insidious pressure from governments. Savings to cash-strapped health and social services are often mooted. The birth of children with the poten-tial of becoming adults with seriously debilitating and costly diseases is frowned upon especially when the technology exists to avoid this scenario. Some govern-ments are careful to disguise the message. Eugenics is a word that sits uncom-fortably within the realms of a civilized society. Recent European history has seen eugenics in action. Many people feel that the continuing striving towards the elim-ination of disabilities through testing and selection is eugenics by the back door.

Some people do not wish to be referred to a genetic centre because it will be entered on their medical records. Many people with sensitive genetic informa-tion are afraid of its misuse by insurance agencies. They are afraid that infor-mation may be disseminated to their disadvantage in applications for life, health or disability insurance. Genetic centres may also put pressure on couples by providing only a limited range of tests and by only offering direct mutation prenatal testing if an at-risk parent has been tested according to the guidelines. One is forced to question such decisions. Surely every person at risk should be given the option of the range of prenatal tests and have the implications explained to them. Individuals should be entitled to decide which test they pre-fer, which risks they wish to take and whether or not they can face, for example, the risk of double bad news.

Genetic centres may also unintentionally put pressure on HD families with-in the framework of their research programmes. For example, a couple may withdraw from prenatal testing and decide to have children that have not been tested. It is important that families do not feel that professionals are critical of their decisions.

5. Other issues

It is clear that although the lay associations have members with a multiplic-ity of views it is generally considered that people should have equal access to the range of services on offer. Although the uptake for tests of all kinds is relatively low this should not be a reason for insufficient funding of these services. It is not the number of prenatal tests but the quality of family planning that counts.

It is important that everyone for whom this is an issue is informed about the available choices. Lay organizations can play an important part in this process. It is essential that all lay associations keep abreast of developments and update their information regularly.

The genetic centres must give information both orally and in writing in order to give couples the opportunity to think, discuss and ask for a second opinion. All relevant options and problems that may arise from tests should be discussed openly and sufficient time must be given to allow for proper understanding. These are complex issues and it is advisable to check what has been understood or misunderstood during the preliminaries of the testing process. Couples must be given the option of referral to another genetic centre if the type of prenatal testing they have chosen is not available. It must be emphasized that the right exists to withdraw from prenatal testing at any time.

Many, but not all, associations believe that prenatal direct mutation testing, without testing the at-risk parent, should be available and therefore this option should be included in the international guidelines (International Huntington Association and World Federation of Neurology, 1994).

It is important that greater awareness, knowledge and understanding of the problems of HD families and other families with hereditary diseases are promoted and disseminated. Everyone should have the right to decide whether or not to raise a family. People at risk of hereditary disease should not be considered as a burden to society. For this generation predictive testing, prenatal testing and now PGD is providing more options. Sadly though, having a choice doesn't necessarily solve anything. These choices are hard choices. We must strive to ensure that people have equal access to these options. If people decide not to avail themselves of new procedures they too must be supported. It is important that we should respect people's decisions, whatever they may be, and strive for a society where all members of it are equally valued, whatever their inheritance.

It would seem that for every problem solved by new tests new ones are created. These are problems for HD families, for geneticists, gynaecologists and healthcare professionals. Each profession has its own ethical and moral codes and responsibilities. From time to time these may seem to conflict with the needs and wishes of the patient. For example, some geneticists may refuse an exclusion test because they believe it is inappropriate for a parent to choose an abortion for a fetus at only 50% risk when a direct test could clarify the status once and for all. It is also true that individual people have their own ethical and moral codes and responsibilities. When different moral stances come into conflict it is important that every effort is made to accommodate the wishes of the individual confronted by hereditary disease within the - confines of the law.

References

Chung, K. (1999) *Designer Myths: The Science, Law and Ethics of Preimplantation Genetic Diagnosis*. Progress Educational Trust, London.

Evers-Kiebooms, G., Swerts, A., Cassiman, J.J. and Van den Berghe, H. (1989) The motivation of at risk individuals and their partners in deciding for or against predictive testing for Huntington's disease. *Clin. Genet.* **35:** 29–40.

International Huntington Association and World Federation of Neurology (1994) Guidelines for the molecular genetics predictive test in Huntington's disease. *Neurology* **44:** 1533–1536.

11

Predictive and prenatal testing for autosomal dominant cerebellar ataxias

Alexandra Dürr and Josué Feingold

1. Introduction

Autosomal dominant cerebellar ataxias (ADCA) are clinically and genetically heterogeneous disorders. Major advances have been made in the diagnosis of ADCA since genetic markers came into use in the 1980s. The subsequent mapping of 16 genes, designated spinocerebellar ataxia (*SCA1–SCA8*, *SCA10–SCA17*), 8 of which have been identified, highlighted their great genetic heterogeneity. The underlying mutations are mostly triplet repeat expansions and the boundaries for genetic testing are well established for the most frequent forms, such as *SCA1*, *–2*, *–3*, *–6* and *–7*. Presymptomatic testing is offered upon request of at-risk persons from ADCA families in which the responsible gene is known, to determine the genetic status of the requester. Recent elucidation of the molecular basis of several ADCA has increased the number of diseases for which at-risk persons can request to know their genetic status. Huntington's disease (HD) represents the first model of direct presymptomatic testing in neurodegenerative disorders and the experience gained since 1993 has allowed the implementation of presymptomatic testing for ADCA in clinical practice. However, although ADCA are rare disorders, the relatively important number of presymptomatic testing requests in these conditions provides interesting insights into the problems raised by presymptomatic testing in neurodegenerative diseases different from HD. This knowledge of demand and outcome of presymptomatic testing in ADCA will help to anticipate the issues of presymptomatic testing in other adult-onset neurodegenerative disorders for which presymptomatic testing will soon be available. As genetic diagnosis becomes available for conditions such as inherited dementias, neuropathies or

Prenatal Testing for Late-Onset Neurogenetic Diseases, edited by G. Evers-Kiebooms, M. W. Zoeteweij and P. S. Harper

neuromuscular disorders, clinicians should be ready to consider presymptomatic testing requests from at-risk individuals and give them the opportunity of an informed choice to take the test or not. The purpose of this chapter is to report the experience of presymptomatic testing in ADCA and to compare it with that in HD.

2. Clinical and molecular features of autosomal dominant cerebellar ataxias

Autosomal dominant cerebellar ataxias are characterized by variable degrees of cerebellar and brainstem dysfunction. Patients usually present with progressive cerebellar gait and the associated signs define three groups of phenotypes according to Harding's clinical classification (Harding, 1993). ADCA type I is the most common group and variably combines cerebellar ataxias and dysarthria with ophthalmoplegia, pyramidal or extrapyramidal signs, amyotrophy and rarely dementia (*Table 1*). ADCA type II combines cerebellar ataxia with macular dystrophy and other neurological signs, whereas type III represents pure cerebellar ataxia with no or very few associated signs. However, the phenotype (e.g. the combination of neurological signs) cannot be predicted from the genotype, except for ADCA type II or SCA7, which is associated with visual loss due to macular degeneration. Even in ADCA type II there are late-onset cases in which visual loss can be missing. Mean age at onset is 35 years but with a wide range, from birth up to 70 years. The disease progression is unremitting and no curative treatment exists today. Psychological support should be part of treatment of these disabling diseases, in addition to medical care, often limited to physiotherapy.

As in HD, a polyglutamine-coding CAG repeat expansion is the responsible mutation for the disease in six of the genes: *SCA1, –2, –3, –6, –7* and *–17*. The disorders caused by these CAG repeat expansion in coding regions of the gene share common properties, important for presymptomatic testing: (i) onset is mostly in adult life; (ii) the disease manifests above a threshold value of CAG repeats on the expanded allele; (iii) the disease course is progressive leading to loss of autonomy and often, death after 5 to 20 years of evolution; (iv) there is a strong negative correlation between the number of CAG repeats on the expanded allele and age at onset; and (v) the repeat sequence is unstable during transmission and has a tendency to increase, particularly in offspring of affected fathers, accounting for the phenomenon of anticipation. Therefore, the larger the repeat, the younger the onset. However, the correlation curves between the size of the expansion and the age at onset are different among SCAs and the important individual variability does not allow one to predict age at onset on the basis of the size of the CAG repeat expansion.

Boundaries between normal and pathological repeats are well defined but they differ among SCAs (*Table 2*). Usually normal and pathological allele ranges do not overlap, except for SCA1 and SCA2. However, in SCA1 and SCA2 most of the normal alleles are interrupted by 1–3 CAT and CAA

Table 1. Clinical and genetic classification of autosomal dominant cerebellar ataxias

Type	Associated signs in addition to cerebellar ataxia	Gene	Locus	Repeat expansion
I	Ophthalmoplegia, optic atrophy, dementia, extrapyramidal signs, amyotrophy	SCA1	6p	Coding CAG
		SCA2	12q	Coding CAG
		SCA3 or Machado-Joseph Disease	14q	Coding CAG
		SCA4	16q	?
		SCA12	5	Non-coding CAG
		SCA14	19q	?
		SCA17 or TBP	6q	Coding CAG
II	Progressive macular dystrophy	SCA7		Coding CAG
III	Pure form	SCA5		?
		SCA6		Coding CAG
		SCA8		CTG?
		SCA11		?
Others	Epilepsy	SCA10		CATTC
	Mental retardation	SCA13		?
	Epilepsy, chorea, dementia	DRPLA		Coding CAG

TBP, TATA box binding protein; DRPLA, dentatorubral-pallidoluysian atrophy.

Table 2. Range of the repeat number in different genetic subtypes of autosomal dominant cerebellar ataxias with coding CAG repeats*

Gene	Range of repeat number		
	Normal	Pathological	Intermediate†
SCA1	6–44	39–83	39–44
SCA2	14–31	32–77	32–33
SCA3	12–44	54–89	
SCA6	7–19	20–30	
SCA7	4–35	37–306	
SCA17 or TBP ‡	25–42	45–63	
DRPLA	7–35	39–88	

*According to Stevanin et al. (2000).
†Sequencing of the CAG repeats in the intermediate range is needed to distinguish between large normal and pathological alleles.
‡Fujiasaki et al. (2001).

respectively, which allows accurate interpretation of the results of molecular analyses (Cancel et al., 1997; Quan et al., 1995).

Other SCA loci are more rare and linkage has been established only in a limited number of families in which indirect predictive testing can be offered. Indirect testing requires an estimation of the risk of recombination between the unknown gene and the markers used for testing to be included in the disclosed result.

Considering the great genetic heterogeneity of ADCA, it is crucial to identify the responsible mutation prior to offering presymptomatic testing in any family. We have encountered at-risk individuals seeking presymptomatic testing for ADCA in which the affected member of their family had negative tests for all known loci, indicating that the family had another form of autosomal dominant cerebellar ataxia for which presymptomatic testing is not yet possible. In other families, all affected members are deceased without prior molecular analyses or DNA banking which also precludes performing presymptomatic testing.

3. Is there a demand for presymptomatic testing in autosomal dominant cerebellar ataxias?

From February 1994 to June 2001, there were 53 requests for presymptomatic testing for at-risk individuals from families with known genotype at our centre of the Hôpital de la Salpêtrière in Paris. The relative frequency of SCA genotypes among candidates for presymptomatic testing is shown in *Table 3* and compared with that of ADCA in the families referred to our diagnostic laboratory. The distribution is similar, even if *SCA1* and *SCA7* are slightly over represented. This could be explained by the fact that *SCA1* was the first gene to be identified for ADCA and by the greater severity of *SCA7* compared with other SCAs because of the presence of vision loss. Given the number of ADCA families tested in our centre, we estimate that there were

Table 3. Comparison of the relative frequency of mutations in *SCA1, -2, -3, -6* and *-7* between families with autosomal dominant cerebellar ataxias and requesters for presymptomatic testing (Hôpital de la Salpêtrière, Paris)

	Relative frequency in families with ADCA (n = 224)	Relative frequency in presymptomatic testing requesters (n = 53)
SCA1	22%	30%
SCA2	22%	15%
SCA3	53%	36%
SCA6	2%	8%
SCA7	1%	11%

approximately 900 individuals at 50% risk and over the age of 18 in these families. To date, approximately 6% of this at-risk population has contacted our centre for information on presymptomatic testing. This is less than for HD, in which a rate of 18% uptake was previously reported in the UK (Harper, 2000). However, presymptomatic testing was initiated earlier for HD than for ADCA and HD families might be better informed about the possibility of presymptomatic testing. Nevertheless, given that a positive diagnosis in our centre is associated with genetic counselling for most patients, it is unlikely that a large proportion of at-risk individuals in our ADCA families are not aware of the existence of presymptomatic testing. A study in two large families with SCA1 prior to the identification of the gene showed that two-thirds of at-risk persons planned to have presymptomatic testing when available (Nance *et al.,* 1994). Our experience shows that, as in HD, the post-gene reality is a lower uptake of presymptomatic testing than anticipated before its availability.

4. Outcome in 53 at-risk persons requesting presymptomatic testing

The procedure in our centre was the same as recommended for HD (International Huntington's Association and World Federation of Neurology, 1994). The step-by-step counselling was performed by the same team as in HD. It included three counselling sessions: the first with the geneticist and neurogeneticist followed, upon request from the at-risk person, by two interviews, one with the psychologist and one with the social worker. The possibility of stopping or postponing testing was always present. Finally, upon request, the at-risk person met the geneticist again to be sampled for molecular analysis with written consent. Disclosure of the result was then completed by follow-up by one of the member of the team chosen by the at-risk person. Follow-up during the first month was systematically proposed but in the long-term it remains each person's decision.

There were 53 at-risk persons asking for presymptomatic testing in our centre. Mean age at contact with the genetic centre for those who asked for presymptomatic testing was 33 ± 10 years, very close to the mean age at onset of the disease. The majority were 50% at risk (n = 48) and the remaining 25%

at risk; as expected by the experience of presymptomatic testing in HD, there were significantly more women than men (35 versus 18) asking for the test and having a test result (21 versus 14), compared with the expected 1 : 1 sex ratio in an autosomal dominant disease. Thirty-five people (66%) requested a result after the presymptomatic testing procedure (*Figure 1*). Fifteen persons did not pursue testing after the first information session and an additional seven withdrew after more counselling but four of the latter seven came back later and obtained their result. Results were disclosed to three individuals and molecular analyses were still underway for four. Considering the high number of drop-outs it seems essential to give time to decide after appropriate information. It would be particularly damaging if all at-risk persons asking for presymptomatic testing were sampled during the first interview because at the end 34% of them would regret knowing their genetic status.

5. What are the motivations and reasons for requesting presymptomatic testing in autosomal dominant cerebellar ataxias?

Although in HD the main reason for presymptomatic testing is the need to know, in our series of at-risk individuals from ADCA kindreds, family planning was the most common motivation to take the test. Fourteen at-risk persons wanted to

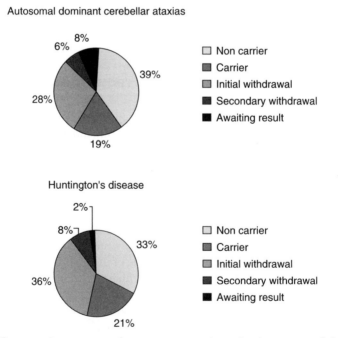

Figure 1. Outcome in requesters for presymptomatic testing in autosomal dominant cerebellar ataxia and Huntington's disease is similar.

have a baby and an additional four came because of an ongoing pregnancy. Only three of the pregnant couples took the test. For 17 individuals the major motivation was to know their own status. The fear of already being affected and believing to be a carrier made 11 persons contact our genetic centre. This is significantly more than in HD because onset in HD is usually very insidious and patients are often unaware of their abnormal movements and of their behavioural changes. In contrast, gait instability as the presenting symptom is usually noticed rapidly after onset by ADCA patients and their relatives. Finally, seven individuals wanted to inform their already born children and to prepare for their own and their children's future. Unfortunately, our series is too small to compare motivations for taking the test according to the genetic subtypes of ADCA.

6. The consequences of presymptomatic testing in autosomal dominant cerebellar ataxias

To date, 31 results have been given: non-carrier for 21 and carrier for 10. Almost half of the persons who had a result (14/31) wished to have a follow-up by one of us. This low proportion is probably due to the fact that testing is a recent practice in these disorders. In HD almost 80% have been followed up in our centre but sometimes only several years after the result. Not surprisingly, a greater proportion of carriers came for follow-up than non-carriers (6/10 versus 8/21). As for HD, coping with carrier and non-carrier status is not always as expected according to the nature of the result: a non-carrier stated '. . . I became someone banal, mortal like everybody. . . .' and a carrier said '. . . finally I do not need to hide anything anymore. . .'. There was no suicide or suicide attempt, but a single carrier underwent depression, which required treatment without hospitalization. The proportion of post-test depression (5%) was similar to that found for presymptomatic testing in HD in our centre. The frequency of catastrophic events has been evaluated in a multicentre study including 175 in 26 countries for presymptomatic testing in HD. Catastrophic events were experienced by 0.97% of at-risk individuals being tested, 85% of which in carriers. Predictive testing for HD may have serious risks, even though the frequency of catastrophic events is lower than previously feared (Almqvist et al., 1999). Although there are close similarities between HD and ADCA, the significantly less frequent past psychiatric history in ADCA (24 versus 6% in our series) may predict that psychiatric consequences of presymptomatic testing will be weaker.

7. Prenatal testing in autosomal dominant cerebellar ataxias

Thirty-four per cent of at-risk individuals requested the test because of a desire for children ($n = 14$) or an ongoing pregnancy ($n = 4$). Interestingly, an ongoing pregnancy was found in six couples but the pregnancy was a situation which urged the presymptomatic testing request only in four. One of the two remaining couples was not considering prenatal testing as an option and in the other the at-risk father decided not to have presymptomatic testing. Among the 10 carriers, 8 were aged under 40 years and 3 of them requested the test to decide for future pregnancies. Finally two couples had five prenatal tests. In one couple the first two prenatal tests resulted in a carrier status for the fetus and were followed by termination of the pregnancy before the third prenatal test with a non-carrier result. In the other couple, who were seen during their first pregnancy, presymptomatic testing was performed after delivery with a carrier result. It was followed by two prenatal tests, with a favorable result the first time but a carrier status of the fetus in the following pregnancy resulting in termination.

8. Conclusion

Predictive testing in ADCA is still part of the genetic predictive protocols, currently being offered within research programmes. As predictive testing is transferred from an academic research context into routine clinical practice, the extensive pre- and post-test counselling is likely to be shortened and multidisciplinary teams reduced because of cost. Our experience at the Salpêtrière Hospital demonstrates that, although the manifestations of the diseases are different, at-risk persons for ADCA do not behave differently from those at risk for HD. The major difference observed to date concerns the most frequent motivation for taking the presymptomatic test: to know their own status in HD but for family planning in ADCA. Time for counselling before taking the test and counsellors' diversity to provide information and to contribute to the maturation of the person's decision seem to us the most essential points. It is important to underline that a significant proportion of at-risk persons choose not to pursue their request for a result. The professionals involved in predictive testing should respect the choice of the at-risk persons and help them make an informed and free choice. The long-term consequences of predictive testing in ADCA are not yet known but there is need for studies which will allow to give a reasonable indication on the type of counselling and the timeframe appropriate for predictive testing protocols.

References

Almqvist, E., Bloch M., Brinkman R., Craufurd D., Hayden M. and the Huntington Disease Collaborative Group (1999) A worldwide assessment of the frequency of suicide, suicide attempts, or psychiatric hospitalization after predictive testing for Huntington's disease. *Am. J. Hum. Genet.* **64:** 1293–1304.

Cancel, G., Dürr, A., Didierjean, O., *et al* (1997) Molecular and clinical correlations in spinocerebellar ataxia 2: a study of 32 families. *Hum. Mol. Genet.* **6:** 709–715.

Fujigasaki, H., Martin, J.J., De Deyn, P.P., Camuzat, A., Deffond, D., Dermaut, B., Van Broeckhoven, C., Dürr, A. and Brice, A. (2001) CAG repeat expansion in the TATA box-binding protein gene causes autosomal dominant cerebellar ataxia. *Brain* **124:** 1939–1947.

Harding, A. (1993) Clinical features and classification of inherited ataxias. *Adv. Neurol.* **61:** 1–14.

Harper P., Lim C., Craufurd D. and the UK Huntington's Disease Prediction Consortium (2000) Ten years of presymtomatic testing for the Huntington's disease: the experience of the UK Huntington's Disease Prediction Consortium. *J. Med. Genet.* **37:** 567–571.

International Huntington's Association and World Federation of Neurology (1994) Guidelines for the molecular genetic predictive test in Huntington's disease. *J. Med. Genet.* **31:** 555–559.

Nance, M., Sevenich, E. and Schut, L. (1994) Knowledge of genetics and attitudes toward genetic testing in two hereditary ataxia (SCA1) kindreds. *Am. J. Med. Genet.* **54:** 242–248.

Quan, F., Janas, J. and Popvich, B.W. (1995) A novel CAG repeat configuration in the *SCA1* gene: implications for the molecular diagnosis of spinocerebellar ataxia type 1. *Hum. Mol. Genet.* **4:** 2411–2413.

Stevanin, G., Durr, A. and Brice, A. (2000) Clinical and molecular advances in autosomal dominant cerebellar ataxias: from genotype to phenotype and physiopathology. *Eur. J. Hum. Genet.* **8:** 4–18.

12

Counselling aspects of prenatal testing for late-onset neurogenetic diseases

David Craufurd

1. Introduction

Huntington's disease (HD) is often used by clinical geneticists as a paradigm for other late-onset inherited disorders, including the many neurodegenerative conditions that have a genetic aetiology. This is partly because HD is among the most common and unpleasant diseases seen in the genetic counselling clinic, and amply illustrates the practical, psychological and social problems facing those who are at risk of inheriting one of these disorders. However, HD was also the first adult-onset human genetic disease for which the responsible gene was initially localized, and then identified, by molecular genetic research methods. Consequently, the practical, ethical and genetic counselling problems arising from the clinical application of this new knowledge in the form of predictive and prenatal genetic testing were first worked out for HD, and the lessons learned have subsequently been modified and applied to other disorders with similar clinical and genetic characteristics. Much of this chapter therefore follows the same convention and focuses on a discussion of the genetic counselling issues associated with prenatal testing for HD, but there are many similar, if much less common, late-onset inherited neurodegenerative disorders for which the same general principles apply.

The experience of being at risk for HD has been vividly described by Wexler (1979). Those with a parent affected by this disorder not only have to live with a 50/50 risk that they will develop the condition themselves, but the fact that onset is usually delayed until the fourth or fifth decade means that they have to make major life decisions concerning education, career, marriage and repro-ductive choices without knowing whether they have inherited the abnormal

Prenatal Testing for Late-Onset Neurogenetic Diseases, edited by G. Evers-Kiebooms, M. W. Zoeteweij and P. S. Harper

gene. Many at-risk individuals find that the uncertainty caused by their genetic risk status makes such decision-making extremely difficult. The discovery of the gene responsible for HD, and the development of techniques such as chorionic villus biopsy (CVB) which allow prenatal sampling of fetal DNA for genetic testing, are major advances which have provided those at-risk with the means to predict in advance whether a particular child is likely to be affected. However, the ability to perform prenatal diagnosis (or strictly speaking, prenatal predictive testing) has also brought new responsibilities and dilemmas for genetic counsellors and their patients. Decisions regarding prenatal testing and the potential termination of high-risk pregnancies are among the most difficult and emotionally charged situations encountered in the genetic clinic, and require great skill and care on the part of the counsellor.

2. Uptake of prenatal testing

Most at-risk individuals requesting adult presymptomatic genetic testing, if they have not already completed their families, mention concern about passing the disorder on to their children as one of the most important reasons for having a predictive test, whereas those who already have children usually say that they wish to provide them with accurate information about their own risk (Bloch et al., 1989; Craufurd, 1989; Meissen et al., 1988; Tibben et al., 1993). Such comments suggest that a significant proportion of people who undergo predictive testing intend to limit the size of their families or refrain from reproduction altogether if the test result is unfavourable, and it is likely that there have always been some at-risk individuals who avoid having children rather than risk the transmission of HD to the next generation of their families. Similar attitudes exist among the general population; for example, a survey examining attitudes to predictive testing among young Belgian women who were not themselves at risk identified 'having more control over the health of offspring' as the most important advantage of genetic counselling (Decruyenaere et al., 1993). However, the uptake of predictive testing in the at-risk population has always been low (Craufurd et al., 1989) and is still no more than about 20% in spite of the widespread availability of direct mutation testing for the past 7 years (Harper et al., 2000). The factors which determine whether or not people request predictive testing are complex and include practical considerations to do with the utility of the test (Evans et al., 2001), personality variables (van der Steenstraten et al., 1994), and individuals' perceptions concerning their ability to cope with the emotional impact of an unfavourable result (Binedell et al., 1998).

In view of the relative importance given to reproductive decision-making by people asked about their reasons for requesting adult predictive testing, it is perhaps surprising that prenatal testing has not been taken up more widely. Full prenatal testing by direct mutation analysis allows couples who want to have children, but are not prepared to risk passing on the abnormal gene, to go ahead with a pregnancy in the certain knowledge that their child will not be

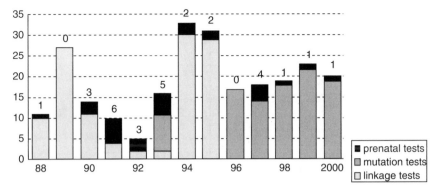

Figure 1. Numbers of prenatal and adult predictive tests for Huntington's disease performed by the North West Regional Genetic Service in Manchester each year (1998–2000).

affected, even if the at-risk parent has had an unfavourable test result. Prenatal exclusion testing provides a solution to this problem for the majority of at-risk individuals who would prefer not to have a predictive test themselves. However, the actual uptake of both types of prenatal test has been very low. This is clearly illustrated in *Fig. 1*, which shows the numbers of predictive and prenatal tests for HD performed each year from 1988 to 2000 by the Regional Genetic Service in Manchester, which serves a population of about 4.5 million in the North West of England. During this 13-year period there were only 28 prenatal tests for HD, compared with a total of 206 adult predictive tests. This figure is consistent with reports in the literature from other centres. Adam *et al.* (1993) reported that during the early years of predictive testing by linkage analysis in Canada, there were 47 pregnancies among the group of patients considering predictive testing; only 14 (30%) requested prenatal testing, whereas 24 did not and a further 9 had no need because their predictive test results put them at low risk. Seven of the 14 decided eventually not to proceed, giving an uptake rate for prenatal testing of just 7/38 (18%) in this group of well-informed individuals who had sought out counselling to discuss genetic testing for themselves. At about the same time, an international survey found that fewer than 250 prenatal tests were performed worldwide between 1986 and 1994, whereas the centres included in the survey performed several thousand predictive tests during the same period (Evers-Kiebooms, 1995). Inspection of the data in *Figure 1* shows no evidence of an increase in the number of prenatal tests per year since the introduction of direct mutation testing, and this is borne out by the results of more recent surveys discussed in detail in Chapter 3.

Understanding the factors which influence decision-making is important for genetic counselling purposes, and there may be many reasons why at-risk couples are not opting for prenatal testing in spite of the potential advantages. If the at-risk parent is already affected or has had an unfavourable predictive test, worry about the future ability of the affected individual to cope with the demands of parenthood, or that personality changes and other behavioural symptoms in the affected parent (Craufurd and Snowden, in press) could have a potential impact

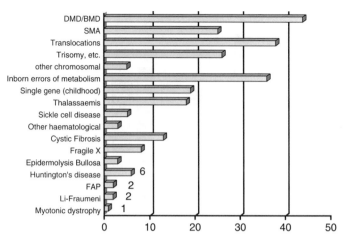

Figure 2. Numbers of prenatal tests for all indications performed by the North West Regional Genetic Service in Manchester during the 3-year period from 1997 to1999.

on the emotional development of the child, may outweigh their concerns about passing on the abnormal gene. In the case of exclusion testing, there is also evidence that many couples do not consider the prospect of their child developing HD in later life to be sufficient justification for terminating a pregnancy at only 50% risk. The emotional trauma associated with terminating a wanted pregnancy is in itself likely to be a major deterrent for many. However, a clue to the most important reason for low uptake of HD prenatal testing can be seen in *Fig. 2*, which shows a breakdown by indication of all the prenatal tests performed by the North West Regional Genetic Service in Manchester during the last 3 years. Almost all these tests were performed because the fetus was at risk of a disorder likely to cause congenital abnormalities or serious illness with a high probability of onset in childhood, whereas fewer than half of 1% were for adult-onset conditions such as HD or inherited cancer syndromes. This may be due to increasing optimism in society at large about the ability of science to develop cures for these disorders in the course of the next few years; alternatively, it may simply reflect a general human tendency to focus more strongly on imminent dangers and threats than those in the more remote future.

3. Direct mutation analysis

The identification of the genetic mutation responsible for HD (Huntington's Disease Collaborative Group, 1993) has greatly simplified genetic testing for this disorder. A single triplet-repeat mutation accounts for all cases of HD, and it is becoming clear that very similar mutations account for a good many other late-onset neurodegenerative disorders as well (David *et al.*, 1997; Kawaguchi *et al.*, 1994; Orr *et al.*, 1993; Sanpei *et al.*, 1996; Zhuchenko *et al.*, 1997). A simple, inexpensive laboratory test using PCR to amplify the DNA sequence containing the mutation can be applied directly to fetal tissue obtained by CVB without the need to culture cells first, or to have previously carried out time-consuming laboratory procedures such as gene sequencing to establish the nature of the mutation carried by the affected members of the family. The advantages of this situation include the ability to perform prenatal testing and obtain a result during the first trimester of pregnancy, allowing termination of pregnancy to be performed using methods which are safer and less distressing for the mother of a high-risk fetus. Early prenatal testing, and if necessary ter-mination of pregnancy, also affords greater privacy for the couple concerned, as does the fact that DNA samples from other family members are no longer necessary, in contrast to earlier methods based on analysis of linked genetic markers. It is also more accurate than testing based on linkage analysis, which involves a margin of error due to the possibility of genetic recombination between the marker and the HD locus, and detection of inconsistent haplo-types due to recombination or other sources of error such as non-paternity is often more difficult with prenatal than predictive testing because of the smaller number of samples usually involved (King *et al.*, 1993).

Although superior in many ways to linkage analysis, direct mutation testing of fetal DNA has the obvious disadvantage that an unfavourable result reveals the at-risk parent to be a carrier of the mutation too. It is therefore most suit-able for testing the offspring of couples where the at-risk partner is already affected, or is known to carry the mutation following a predictive test. However, it is quite unusual for couples to plan a pregnancy after one of them has become symptomatic, perhaps because of the concerns mentioned above about their likely capacity to fulfil parental responsibilities until the child is old enough to be fully independent. The low uptake of predictive testing among at-risk adults means that many of those who would consider prenatal testing will not have had a test themselves, and would prefer not to do so. A direct prenatal test in these circumstances means that in the event of an unfavourable result the at-risk parent will discover his or her own genetic status, and be obliged to face up to the personal implications of this at the same time as coping with the termin-ation of a planned and wanted pregnancy. Furthermore, the need to obtain a result in time for a first-trimester termination of pregnancy means that a decision about whether to go ahead with prenatal testing often has to be made very quickly. The widely accepted ethical guidelines governing adult predictive testing for HD (International Huntington Association and World Federation of Neurology Research Group on Huntington's Chorea, 1994) recommend a minimum of two genetic counselling sessions to prepare for a decision about predictive testing, separated by an adequate interval for reflection on the issues involved, but adherence to these guidelines in the context of prenatal testing is impossible if the process has not started before the pregnancy is diagnosed.

4. Prenatal exclusion testing

Prenatal exclusion testing provides a way for prospective parents who are them-selves at 50% risk to ensure that their offspring are at low risk, without having to find out whether they carry the HD mutation themselves (Hayden *et al.*, 1987; Quarrell *et al.*, 1987). The technique involves the use of genetic markers closely linked to HD to determine whether the HD allele inherited by the fetus from its affected parent came from the affected or unaffected grandparent. A fetus with the haplotype of markers originating from the affected grandparent inherits the same 50% risk as the intervening parent, and in these circumstances the pregnancy would be terminated. Conversely, a fetus inheriting the marker haplotype originating with the unaffected grandparent has a very low risk. Even if the fetus does inherit the high-risk haplotype, the test result does not change the 50% risk for the intervening parent, a point which many couples find difficult to grasp (Adam *et al.*, 1993; Tyler *et al.*, 1990). It is therefore very important for genetic counsellors to ensure that the implications of the test have been fully explained and understood, in order to avoid a situation in which one or other of the parents erroneously believes that because the prenatal test was unfavourable, the at-risk individual must inevitably carry the mutant gene.

Exclusion testing would be the ideal solution for couples who want to have a prenatal test without changing the at-risk status of the at-risk person, were it not for the prospect of terminating a pregnancy with only a 50% risk of being affected. Although some have questioned the ethical basis for selective termination of pregnancy in these circumstances (Post, 1992), most people would probably regard the prospect of developing HD as sufficient justification for this course of action, especially when this is seen in the context that roughly one in five pregnancies in the UK currently end in termination (Paxman, 1999). The main difficulty in this situation arises from the fact that these are wanted pregnancies, and the decision to terminate them usually involves a considerable degree of emotional anguish and distress for the parents involved. It is therefore not unusual for couples faced with an unfavourable exclusion test result to make a last-minute request for definitive mutation analysis in the hope that this will provide a reprieve, even though they had previously taken a firm decision not to have a predictive test themselves. In some cases this is deliberately planned in advance as a stepwise procedure involving a preliminary exclusion test, to be followed by a definitive mutation test for themselves and the fetus if the initial exclusion test proves unfavourable (Fahy *et al.*, 1989). Although this approach removes any danger of terminating an unaffected pregnancy, it has the drawback that an unfavourable result leaves the at-risk parent to cope with the loss of a wanted pregnancy at the same time as coming to terms with the personal implications of an unfavourable predictive test result for which neither party has been adequately prepared. Although it is unsatisfactory in many ways, this exclusion-definitive approach not only avoids the need to terminate a possibly unaffected pregnancy, but has the advantage that there is only a 25% risk of bad news, compared with a 50% risk if the at-risk parent has a predictive test first. All these options need to be discussed with the couple before a decision to undergo prenatal testing is made, but it is easy for someone previously unfamiliar with the issues involved to become confused, and this is not a process that can be rushed. Even if there is some urgency to make a decision so that a CVB can be arranged, it may be appropriate to arrange a further appointment after 2 or 3 days so that the couple have time to reflect on their decision and seek further information or clarification before finally making up their minds how to proceed.

Although the decision to terminate a pregnancy can be a very difficult one for prospective parents in these circumstances, the alternative decision to continue with a pregnancy following an unfavourable prenatal test raises even more difficult issues. Even an unfavourable exclusion test means that the fetus has the marker haplotype inherited from the affected grandparent, and shares the same 50% risk of HD as the intervening parent. Unless the pregnancy is terminated, the subsequent appearance of symptoms in the at-risk parent would immediately reveal the child to be a carrier of the HD mutation too, and amounts to a predictive test carried out without reference to the wishes of the child. The low uptake of adult predictive testing for HD suggests that a large majority of at-risk individuals would prefer not to have this information. Parents sometimes request predictive testing for their children, but as there is currently nothing that can be done to delay or prevent the onset of the disease in known gene carriers, there is a consensus among clinical geneticists that predictive genetic testing of children for late-onset diseases such as HD is unethical (Clinical Genetics Society, 1994). Consequently, it is inappropriate to offer prenatal testing if the at-risk couple do not have a clear intention to terminate the pregnancy in the event of an unfavourable result (Quarrell et al., 1987), and it is important that this issue is addressed during counselling. There will inevitably be instances in which a couple start out with the intention to terminate the pregnancy after an unfavourable result, but subsequently change their minds (Tolmie et al., 1995); however, this situation is less likely to occur if the individuals concerned have confronted the possibility of an unfavourable result and thought carefully about their reaction to it, rather than simply putting off a decision until later in the hope of a favourable outcome.

5. Implications for existing children

One of the most difficult and complex issues arising from prenatal testing concerns the situation of existing and subsequent children. In the case of a couple who already have one or more at-risk children and are contemplating a prenatal test for a new pregnancy, the decision to proceed with testing has the potential to create a family in which some of the children are at risk, whereas others are not. It may be very difficult to prevent this knowledge from subtly affecting the parents' attitudes to the children, with unpredictable effects on their emotional development. Eventually, the children will have to be told the truth about their family history, thereby creating the possibility of family divisions and relationship problems later on.

This scenario is probably fairly uncommon, because prenatal testing has been available for many years and couples who have already had children without tests are relatively unlikely to request one now unless they have only just become aware of their at-risk status. However, a similar problem applies to any subsequent pregnancies. Having once had a child with a low risk of HD following prenatal testing, it would be impossible not to follow the same course of action in any subsequent pregnancy without creating exactly the same difficulties as described above. Furthermore, many couples find that having once terminated a pregnancy after an unfavourable prenatal test, it is difficult to adopt a different course in any subsequent pregnancies. The emotional trauma associated with multiple terminations of much-wanted pregnancies can be very hard to bear, but the alternative of going ahead with an untested, at-risk pregnancy may be impossible because of a moral obligation to the earlier children. The initial decision to undergo prenatal testing therefore has implications which stretch well beyond the existing pregnancy, and it is important for the genetic counsellor to make sure the couple have considered this before making up their minds.

6. Sex of the at-risk parent

Another potential difficulty associated with prenatal testing for dominantly inherited late-onset disorders such as HD stems from the fact that with this mode of inheritance either parent can be the one at risk, whereas much of the practical and emotional burden of the test procedure falls on the female partner. This is quite different from prenatal testing for recessive or X-linked disorders, where the mother is always at least partly responsible for the genetic risk to the fetus. There is no doubt that the termination of a wanted pregnancy for genetic reasons is emotionally traumatic for both of the parents, who often experience feelings of guilt about their decision, and sometimes a period of depression afterwards (Blumberg et al., 1975; Donnai et al., 1981; White-van Mourik et al., 1992). However, distress following a miscarriage or genetic termination of pregnancy often reveals itself in different ways in males and females; such differences can lead to misunderstandings, and sometimes impose considerable strains on the parents' relationship.

The situation of a couple requesting prenatal testing because the male partner is at 50% risk for HD or a similar dominantly inherited neurogenetic disorder is therefore particularly vulnerable to tensions and pressures of this sort. The female partner of the at-risk individual in such cases is likely to have much less experience and understanding of the emotional and practical burdens imposed by the disease, and may never have received genetic counselling. She may have only recently become aware of the genetic risk to her children, with less time to come to terms with the situation or to prepare for the decisions to be made. It is all too easy for grief and guilt relating to the termination of a high-risk pregnancy in these circumstances to turn into anger and recrimination, especially after a series of unfavourable prenatal tests. It is also possible that the male partner may experience greater feelings of guilt and responsibility about the distress experienced by his spouse if the prenatal test is performed because of his own family history, and suffer a loss of self-esteem as a consequence. Conversely, he may feel rejected or stigmatized if his partner is the one most in favour of prenatal testing.

7. Genetic counselling

Prenatal testing for HD and related neurogenetic disorders presents several difficulties for the genetic counsellor. First, there is the complexity of the choice facing a couple in this situation, and the difficulty of explaining all the potential consequences of these choices in a way which is intelligible to individuals who are unfamiliar with both the methodology and the problems associated with prenatal diagnosis. Second, there is the importance to the couple of the decision to be made, and the emotional trauma surrounding termination of a pregnancy under these circumstances. As noted above, prenatal testing could potentially have long-term consequences for family relationships. Furthermore, many people have strongly held religious or ethical views about abortion, and it is important, but not at all easy, to help at-risk couples arrive at a fully informed decision which is appropriate to their situation, consistent with their own beliefs and values, and independent of the pressures which may be exerted on them by families, friends and society in general. Achieving this takes time.

Unfortunately, time is a commodity that is often in short supply where prenatal testing is concerned. Although the development of CVB has brought undoubted benefits in the sense that earlier prenatal testing allows any subsequent termination of pregnancy to be carried out during the first trimester, it has the drawback for the genetic counsellor that there is now a much shorter interval between the diagnosis of pregnancy and the test procedure itself. By the time a couple reach the genetic counselling clinic there may be very little time for them to explore the options open to them, understand the potential ramifications of each, and arrive at an informed decision. Much of the available time can be taken up with practical issues such as arranging an ultrasound scan to confirm the dates of the pregnancy, or approaching the parents of the at-risk partner to obtain DNA samples for use in prenatal exclusion testing. In the case of exclusion testing, the problem of identifying an informative marker for linkage analysis sometimes involves a considerable amount of work for the laboratory, and can be very time-consuming. The situation is especially difficult if the pregnancy is unplanned or unexpected.

The solution to this problem lies mainly in the timing of genetic counselling (Harper, 1998). Many of these difficulties can be avoided altogether if the couple have already been seen for genetic counselling prior to conception, and have had a previous opportunity to think through their attitude to both adult and prenatal predictive testing. It is much easier to make an objective decision about the advantages and drawbacks of both these procedures *before* a pregnancy occurs, and it is likely that thoughtful preparation for prenatal testing helps to diminish the emotional trauma associated with an unfavourable outcome. However, the need to arrange for genetic counselling to take place before conception has considerable implications for the organization of genetic services. Growing public and professional awareness about molecular genetics and the availability of genetic testing has unfortunately created a situation in which many patients assume this to be the main purpose of genetic counselling, and it is becoming increasingly common to be told by general practitioners that they did not refer an at-risk person to the genetic clinic because the individual concerned had decided not to have a predictive test. Clinical geneticists have much to offer to those at risk of late-onset neurogenetic disorders in addition to predictive testing, but the counselling needs of the at-risk person vary considerably at different stages in life. In an ideal world, services should be organized in such a way that once an at-risk individual has been seen in the genetic clinic, he or she can access further information and support at the time when it is most appropriate, rather than viewing genetic counselling as a 'one-off' activity.

One possible solution to this problem, at least for late-onset dominant disorders such as HD, lies in the development of genetic registers (Dean *et al.*, 2000; Emery *et al.*, 1978). An example of this approach is the Family Genetic Register Service in Manchester, which was set up with the twin aims of providing long-term support and follow-up to families at risk of several dominant or X-linked disorders including HD, and of extending the offer of genetic counselling to at-risk individuals in these families who may not otherwise have been aware of their risk or of the availability and potential benefits of genetic counselling. Once an individual has been seen in the genetic counselling clinic and has consented to inclusion on the register, he or she is contacted annually by letter and asked to return a form designed to ensure that contact details remain up to date; the form includes an opportunity for the patient to request a further appointment if required. The intention is that an at-risk person who was originally seen as a young adult, for example, following the diagnosis of his affected parent, will be encouraged to request further counselling at significant life stages such as when considering marriage or planning to start a family. Individuals on the register are also encouraged to pass on the offer of genetic counselling to other family members who might benefit from this, and a reminder is included in their annual recall letter if there are known to be at-risk relatives who have not yet been seen. A recent study looking at the views of genetic clinic patients with a family history of Duchenne and Becker muscular dystrophy, myotonic dystrophy or balanced chromosome translocations found that this more proactive approach to genetic counselling is highly acceptable to the at-risk individuals themselves and reaches a significantly greater proportion of at-risk family members than more conventional approaches to service delivery (Kerzin-Storrar *et al.*, submitted; Wright *et al.*, submitted).

8. Conclusion

Experience to date with those late-onset inherited disorders such as HD and some inherited cancer syndromes for which genetic testing is currently possible suggests that relatively few at-risk couples take advantage of the opportunity for prenatal testing. The low uptake of prenatal testing for these disorders contrasts with much higher rates for genetic disorders entailing a risk of congenital abnormalities or serious illness in childhood. Nevertheless, there is no doubt that prenatal testing remains a valuable option for some at-risk couples, but can give rise to practical, emotional and ethical difficulties that present considerable challenges for the genetic counsellor.

References

Adam, S., Wiggins, S., Whyte, P., et al (1993) Five year study of prenatal testing for Huntington's disease: demand, attitudes and psychological assessment. *J. Med. Genet.* **30:** 549–556.

Binedell, J., Soldan, J.R. and Harper, P.S. (1998) Predictive testing for Huntington's disease: II. Qualitative findings from a study of uptake in South Wales. *Clin. Genet.* 489–496.

Bloch, M., Fahy, M., Fox, S. and Hayden, M.R. (1989) Predictive testing for Huntington's disease: II. Demographic characteristics, life-style patterns, attitudes and psychosocial assessments of the first fifty one test candidates. *Am. J. Med. Genet.* **32:** 217–224.

Blumberg, B.D., Golbus, M.S. and Hanson, K.H. (1975) The psychological sequelae of abortion performed for a genetic indication. *Am. J. Obstet. Gynaecol.* **122:** 799–808.

Clinical Genetics Society (1994) Report of the Working Party on the genetic testing of children. *J. Med. Genet.* **31:** 785–797.

Craufurd, D. (1989) Progress and problems in Huntington's disease. *Int. Rev. Psychiat.* **1:** 249–258.

Craufurd, D., Dodge, A., Kerzin-Storrar, L. and Harris, R. (1989) Uptake of presymptomatic predictive testing for Huntington's disease. *Lancet* **ii:** 603–605.

Craufurd, D. and Snowden, J.S. Neuropsychological and neuropsychiatric aspects of Huntington's disease. In: *Huntington's Disease*, 3rd edn (eds G. Bates, P.S. Harper and L. Jones) (in press).

David, G., Abbas, N., Stevanin, G., et al (1997) Cloning of the SCA7 gene reveals a highly unstable CAG repeat expansion. *Nat. Genet.* **17:** 65–70.

Dean, J.C.S., Fitzpatrick, D.R., Farnden, P.A. et al. (2000) Genetic registers in clinical practice: a survey of UK clinical geneticists. *J. Med. Genet.* **37:** 636–640.

Decruyenaere, M., Evers-Kiebooms, G. and van den Berghe, H. (1993) Perception of predictive testing for Huntington's disease by young women: preferring uncertainty to certainty? *J. Med. Genet.* **30:** 557–561.

Donnai, P., Charles, N.and Harris, R. (1981) Attitudes of patients after 'genetic' termination of pregnancy. *BMJ* **282:** 621–622.

Emery, A.E.H., Brough, C., Crawfurd, M., Harper, P., Harris, R. and Oakshott, G. (1978) A report on genetic registers. *J. Med. Genet.* **15:** 435–442.

Evans, J.P., Skrzynia, C. and Burke, W. (2001) The complexities of predictive genetic testing. *BMJ* **322:** 1052–1056.

Evers-Kiebooms, G. (1995) Data presented to 16th international meeting of the World Federation of Neurology Research Group on Huntington's disease, Leuven, Belgium, July 1995.

Fahy, M., Robbins, C., Bloch, M., Turnell, R.W. and Hayden, M.R. (1989). Different options for prenatal testing for Huntington's disease using DNA probes. *J. Med. Genet.* **26:** 353–357.

Harper, P.S. (1998). *Practical Genetic Counselling*, 5th edn. Reed Educational and Professional Publishing, Oxford, pp. 103–104.

Harper, P.S., Lim, C., Craufurd, D., on behalf of the UK Huntington's Disease Prediction Consortium (2000) Ten years of presymptomatic testing for Huntington's disease: the experience of the UK Huntington's Disease Prediction Consortium. *J. Med. Genet.* **37:** 567–571.

Hayden, M.R., Hewitt, J, Kastelein, JJ, Langlois, S., Wilson, R.D., Fox, S., Hilbert, C. and Bloch, M. (1987) First-trimester prenatal diagnosis for Huntington's disease with DNA probes. *Lancet* **I:** 1284–1285.

Huntington's Disease Collaborative Research Group (1993) A novel gene containing a trinucleotide repeat that is unstable and expanded on Huntington's disease chromosomes. *Cell* **72:** 971–983.

International Huntington Association and World Federation of Neurology Research Group on Huntington's Chorea (1994) Guidelines for the molecular genetics predictive test in Huntington's disease. *Neurology* **44:** 1533–1536.

Kawaguchi, Y., Okamoto, T., Taniwaki, M., *et al* (1994) CAG expansions in a novel gene for Machado-Joseph disease at chromosome 14q32.1. *Nat. Genet.* **8**: 221–228.

Kerzin-Storrar, L., Wright, C., Williamson, P., Fryer, A., Njindou, A., Quarrell, O., Donnai, D. and Craufurd, D. Comparison of genetic services with and without genetic registers: access and attitudes to genetic counselling services among relatives of genetic clinic patients. *J. Med. Genet.* (submitted).

King, T.M., Brandt, J. and Meyers, D.A. (1993) Effect of laboratory or clerical error on presymptomatic risk calculations for Huntington disease: a simulation study. *Am. J. Med. Genet.* **46**: 154–158.

Meissen, G.J., Myers, R.H., Mastromauro, C.A., Koroshetz, W.J., Klinger, K.W., Farrer, L.A., Watkins, P.A., Gusella, J.F., Bird, E.D. and Martin, J.B. (1988) Predictive testing for Huntington's disease with use of a linked DNA marker. *N. Engl. J. Med.* **318**: 535–542.

Orr, H.T., Chung, M.-Y., Banfi, S., Kwiatkowski, T.J., Servadio, A., Beaudet, A.L., McCall, A.E., Duvick, L.A., Ranum, L.P.W. and Zoghbi, H.Y. (1993) Expansion of an unstable trinucleotide CAG repeat in spinocerebellar ataxia type 1. *Nat. Genet.* **4**: 221–226.

Paxman, J. (1999) *The English*. Penguin Books, London, p. 101.

Post, S.G. (1992) Huntington's disease: prenatal screening for late onset disease. *J. Med. Ethics* **18**: 75–78.

Quarrell, O.W, Meredith, A.L., Tyler, A., Youngman, S., Upadhyaya, M. and Harper, P.S. (1987) Exclusion testing for Huntington's disease in pregnancy with a closely linked DNA marker. *Lancet* **i**: 1281–1283.

Sanpei, K., Takano, H., Igarashi, S., *et al* (1996) Identification of the spinocerebellar ataxia type 2 gene using a direct identification of repeat expansion and cloning technique, DIRECT. *Nat. Genet.* **14**: 277–284.

Tibben, A., Frets, P.G., v.d.Kamp, JJP., Niermeijer, M.F., Vegter-v.d. Vlis, M., Roos, R.A.C., Rooymans, H.G.M., v. Ommen, G.-J.B. and Verhage, F. (1993) On attitudes and appreciation 6 months after predictive DNA testing for Huntington disease in the Dutch program. *Am. J. Med. Genet.* **48**: 103–111.

Tolmie, JL., Davidson, H.R., May, H.M., McIntosh, K., Paterson, JS. and Smith, B. (1995) The prenatal exclusion test for Huntington's disease: experience in the west of Scotland. *J. Med. Genet.* **32**: 97–101.

Tyler, A., Quarrell, O.W., Lazarou, L.P., Meredith, A.L. and Harper, P.S. (1990) Exclusion testing in pregnancy for Huntington's disease. *J. Med. Genet.* **27**: 488–495.

van der Steenstraten, I.M., Tibben, A., Roos, R.A., van de Kamp, J.J. and Niermeijer, M.F. (1994) Predictive testing for Huntington's disease: nonparticipants compared with participants in the Dutch programme. *Am. J. Hum. Genet.* **55**: 618–625.

Wexler, N.S. (1979). Genetic 'Russian roulette': the experience of being at risk for Huntington's disease. In: *Genetic Counselling: Psychological Dimensions* (ed. S. Kessler). Academic Press, New York, pp. 119–220.

White-van Mourik, M.C.A., Connor, J.M. and Ferguson-Smith, M.A. (1992) The psychosocial sequelae of a second-trimester termination of pregnancy for fetal abnormality. *Prenatal Diagn.* **12**: 189–204.

Wright, C., Kerzin-Storrar, L., Williamson, P., Fryer, A., Njindou, A., Quarrell, O., Donnai, D. and Craufurd, D. Comparison of genetic services with and without genetic registers: knowledge, adjustment and attitudes about genetic counselling among probands referred to three regional genetic clinics in the north west of England (submitted).

Zhuchenko, O., Bailey, J., Bonnen, P., Ashizawa, T., Stockton, D.W., Amos, C., Dobyns, W.B., Subramony, S.H., Zoghbi, H.Y. and Cheng Chi Lee (1997) Autosomal dominant cerebellar ataxia (SCA6) associated with small polyglutamine expansions in the α_{1A}-voltage-dependent calcium channel. *Nat. Genet.* **15**: 62–69.

13

Predictive and prenatal testing for late-onset neurogenetic diseases in North America

Martha A. Nance

1. Introduction

Predictive genetic testing for Huntington's disease (HD) has been performed in the US since the mid-1980s, following the discovery of DNA markers genetically linked to the HD gene. However, widespread use of predictive gene tests for adult-onset neurogenetic disorders did not begin until the 1990s, when the identification of the HD gene and several hereditary ataxia genes permitted individuals to undergo simple and accurate blood tests without requiring multiple family members to participate in the testing process. Centres in both the US and Canada, as in Europe, have attempted to assess the effects of and improve upon the use of this new clinical technology by forming consortia of involved individuals, laboratories and clinical centres. This chapter focuses on the experiences of two such groups, the US Huntington Disease Genetic Testing Group (US HD GTG) and the Ataxia Molecular Diagnostic Testing Group (AMDTG), but will also review the contributions of the Canadian Collaborative Study of Predictive Testing for Huntington Disease and of other individual investigators in Canada, the US and Mexico.

2. Uptake of predictive and prenatal testing for Huntington's disease and ataxia

For many reasons, when widespread predictive and prenatal genetic testing for HD became a possibility, both national (Huntington's Disease Society of

Prenatal Testing for Late-Onset Neurogenetic Diseases, edited by G. Evers-Kiebooms, M. W. Zoeteweij and P. S. Harper
©2002 BIOS Scientific Publishers Ltd, Oxford

America) and international (International Huntington Association/World Federation of Neurology) organizations moved quickly to establish guidelines for the performance of this novel clinical procedure (Anonymous, 1994; Huntington's Disease Society of America, 1994). Much of the early work on the effects of predictive testing on tested individuals, as well as clarification of technical issues related to the diagnostic assay itself, was reported by the Canadian Collaborative Study of Predictive Testing in HD (Andrew *et al.*, 1994; Babul *et al.*, 1993; Benjamin *et al.*, 1994; Copley *et al.*, 1995; Hayden *et al.*, 1995; Lawson *et al.*, 1996). Early research at Johns Hopkins University on the effects of predictive testing on individuals and their close relationships also contributed significantly to the tenor of the guidelines (Codori and Brandt, 1994; Codori *et al.*, 1994; Quaid and Wesson, 1995). Attitudes toward the use of predictive and prenatal testing for HD, as well as molecular genetic characteristics were also studied, somewhat later, in Mexico (Alonso *et al.*, 1997; Alonso Vilatela *et al.*, 1999).

By 1996, when the US HD GTG formed under this name, 65 HD 'predictive testing centres', providing the genetic, psychological, and neurological services outlined in the HDSA and IHA/WFN guidelines, had come into existence in the US. At that time, 26 molecular diagnostic laboratories offered an assay of the CAG repeat in the *IT–15* gene as a clinical service. According to GeneTests™ (www.genetests.org), in 2001, 34 different US laboratories offer genetic testing for HD, and at least 25 offer tests for one or more of the spinocerebellar ataxia genes (*SCA1*, *–2*, *–3*, *–6*, *–7*, *–8*, *–10*, *–12*, *DRPLA*, Friedreich's ataxia). Whereas predictive genetic testing for HD in the US still remains relatively restricted to one of the (now) 70 predictive testing centres that offer genetic counselling, psychological support and neurological expertise in HD, no similar restrictions exist for the hereditary ataxias. Prenatal testing for any of the disorders is typically offered by an obstetrician in consultation with a genetic counsellor, and is likely not to involve a specialized predictive testing centre. Because there is no requirement for reporting of prenatal or predictive tests, and participation in the consortia is voluntary for both clinical centres and laboratories, it is certain that the ascertainment of cases by both the US HD GTG and the AMDTG is incomplete.

In the US, 63 of 65 existing predictive testing centres responded to a 1996 survey, which showed that the centres combined had performed 1419 predictive tests by a direct assay of the *IT–15* gene since 1993 – 57% with normal results, 40% showing gene expansions, and slightly less than 3% with 'intermediate' results. Thirty-one centres have continued to provide annual accounts of tests performed; these centres reported a rather constant combined total number of 300–350 predictive tests each year from 1995 to 1999 (Nance *et al.*, 1999). Recognizing that the 2000 survey included slightly less than half of the total number of centres but most of the high-volume ones, and that some patients are being tested outside of predictive testing centres, one can estimate that about 600–750 predictive tests are carried out in the US each year. If current estimates that there are 150 000 Americans with a 50% risk of carrying the HD gene are correct, then fewer than 0.5% of the US at-risk population undergoes predictive testing each year. This figure, albeit a rather loose estimate, is substantially less than the predictive testing rate reported by the UK Consortium (Harper *et al.*, 2000) and elsewhere. The US HD GTG 2000 survey confirmed that in the US, as elsewhere, more women than men undergo predictive testing, by a ratio of close to 60/40. Over one-third of those tested are between the ages of 30 and 39, and 85% are aged between 20 and 49. Ninety-six per cent are of Caucasian descent.

In 1996, the year for which the US HD GTG had the most complete reporting, the 63 responding centres reported a combined total of 14 prenatal tests for the 3 years covered in the survey. Although this number may underestimate the total number of prenatal tests carried out in the US, as there is no requirement for prenatal testing to be done in an HD predictive testing centre, ascertainment of cases through testing laboratories at the same time yielded a similar figure. In 2000, 31 centres reported a total of 38 prenatal tests from 1996 to 1999 (a range of 8–12 per year for all the centres combined), reiterating the impression of a low uptake of this service. Preimplantation testing has been discussed in the US and elsewhere (Braude *et al.*, 1998; Schulman and Black, 1997; Schulman *et al.*, 1996), but has only been documented in one US report (Stern *et al.*, 2000). In Canada, a similar low uptake of prenatal testing was documented prior to the availability of a direct gene test (Adam *et al.*, 1993).

A 1998 survey of the AMDTG showed a total of 2240 ataxia gene tests performed by 12 laboratories for all indications, with 94.6% of all tests yielding normal results. Only 11 predictive tests and 1 prenatal test were reported, suggesting for this group of disorders a low uptake rate similar to that seen for HD (Potter *et al.*, 1998, 2000).

3. Issues in predictive and prenatal testing

3.1 Issues in the diagnostic laboratory

One of the first problems identified by the US HD GTG in 1996 was the definition of the boundaries of 'normal', 'expanded' and 'intermediate' CAG repeat lengths. Among the 16 reporting laboratories, the boundaries of the 'intermediate' result range extended to as low as 30 CAG repeats and as high as 41 CAG repeats, and alleles within the laboratory-defined intermediate range accounted for 2.5% of all upper allele sizes reported by the laboratories. Concern about this problem led to the formation of an American Society of Human Genetics/American College of Medical Genetics *ad hoc* committee, which published a definition of diagnostic boundaries, based on a review of the available literature combined with the experience of the US HD GTG (ACMG/ASHG HD Genetic Testing Working Group, 1998). In this review, CAG repeat lengths of 27–35 were considered to be normal but 'mutable', meaning that CAG repeat numbers in this range had been reported in an asymptomatic parent of an affected 'new mutation' case but not in any well-documented case of symptomatic HD. Repeat lengths of 36–39 repeats were considered to be abnormal, or capable of causing HD, but 'incompletely penetrant', because one or more asymptomatic elderly individuals with repeat lengths in that range had been reported. Repeat lengths of 40 or more were abnormal and essentially fully penetrant within a normal life expectancy. Others have used 42 CAG repeats as the boundary beyond which penetrance is complete (Brinkman et al., 1997).

Technical concerns about laboratory methodology for the HD gene assay are relatively minor; laboratories use methods that distinguish the CAG repeat sequence from the adjacent CCG repeat (Andrew et al., 1994). Some laboratories are not skilled in the use of Southern blot techniques that might be necessary to identify very large repeat lengths associated with very early disease onset (Nance et al., 1999), but referral to other laboratories is possible.

Result interpretation and technical performance have been a major focus of the AMDTG. Happily, proficiency testing for SCA1, –2, –3, –6, –7 and DRPLA showed uniform reporting of allele sizes among laboratories despite some variations in testing methodologies (Potter et al., 2000). Concerns were raised about the interpretation of 'intermediate' range alleles for SCA1, SCA2 and SCA7, and about the possibility that very large SCA2 and SCA7 alleles could be missed using standard PCR-based methodology. A study by the same group of laboratories performing Friedreich's ataxia gene tests found that only two-thirds of reporting laboratories obtained results that were categorically the same as those of the reference laboratory for all four test samples. Most, but not all, of the variances were in distinguishing normal alleles from 'premutation' alleles, and categorical differences appeared to relate to variations in technique rather than to the use of different diagnostic boundaries in reporting (Wick et al., 1999).

Another area of concern for molecular diagnostic laboratories is patenting of gene tests. If a commercial laboratory or entity acquires and enforces a patent for a particular assay, it may preclude the refinement of procedures and interpretations that comes with the shared experience of a group of practitioners. In the case of the hereditary ataxias, a single sample is often subjected efficiently to a multiplexed array of tests; exclusive patenting or licensing of ataxia gene tests could easily increase the cost of or limit access to such gene test panels.

3.2 Predictive testing of children

Predictive testing of juveniles is strongly discouraged in the US, as elsewhere, because the potential adverse psychosocial consequences are relatively higher for children than adults and are not balanced by any medical benefits (American Society of Human Genetics Board of Directors and The American College of Medical Genetics Board of Directors, 1995). In addition, as only a small proportion of at-risk adults in the US choose to undergo predictive testing, it is likely that a parent who requests a predictive test for his or her child is requesting something that the child would not want.

HD predictive testing centres are uniform in their refusal to perform predictive tests on children, but have often been involved in diagnostic testing situations. The US HD GTG found that one-quarter of children tested for 'diagnostic' purposes did not have HD gene expansions, and that 3/44 had gene expansions that appeared inconsistent with the apparent onset age (e.g. a child diagnosed with autism at age 5 who had 43 CAG repeats) (Nance *et al.*, 1997). CAG repeat numbers below 45 were not identified in juvenile-onset cases, either in this series or in the prior literature. This experience reiterates the importance of thorough clinical evaluation prior to gene testing, even in the presence of neurologic or psychiatric symptoms.

3.3 Anonymous testing

A small proportion of individuals requesting genetic predictive testing in the US have an exceptional desire to maintain privacy, and request 'anonymous' testing. The US HD GTG reviewed, by interview with the responsible geneticist or genetic counsellor, 18 cases of anonymous testing (Visintainer *et al.*, 2001). In the absence of any defined protocol for anonymity, and confronted with varying requests from the patients, the counsellors described an interesting range of experiences. Some patients were previously known to the counsellor, and were happy to provide a detailed family history, but simply wanted the blood sample sent to the laboratory with a pseudonym. At the other extreme were patients who would not provide any personal information or family history, who made payments for testing through a third party, and who would not allow the counsellor to initiate any telephone or written contact. The former was termed 'pseudonymous' testing, whereas the latter is closer to a truly 'anonymous' testing situation. Most patients fell somewhere in the middle of this continuum. The more anonymous the testing situation, the more difficulty the counsellors had completing their usual tasks of documenting the family history (although some patients who would not provide their own names were willing to provide names of affected relatives!) and establishing a therapeutic rapport prior to proceeding with the gene test. Anonymous testing patients were predominantly male, and the reasons for anonymous testing were more often related to career or social concerns than to insurance concerns (e.g. some of these individuals worked in the health care or biomedical science fields, or held positions of social prominence in their community).

Several unresolved issues were identified in this study. Most of the counsellors interviewed felt that it remained important to have face-to-face contact with the patient, but found that they had to negotiate with the patient, and clarify in their own minds, which aspects of the standard counselling process they would not deviate from, and which rules could be bent, and to understand why the patient perceived any advantages from anonymous testing (Uhlmann *et al.*, 1996). This negotiation process significantly increased the time that the counsellor spent on the case. Although all counsellors required the patient to sign a consent, most allowed the patient to use a pseudonym on the consent document, raising issues about the consent process as well as the validity of a pseudonymous consent (Sharpe, 1994). In a previous case report from Canada, a concern was articulated that individuals requesting anonymous testing might be more likely than others to experience emotional distress, and that provision of adequate medical or psychiatric care is compromised in the anonymous setting (Burgess *et al.*, 1998). Given the difficulty that the counsellors had in establishing a supportive relationship with these patients, and the challenges of providing ongoing treatment to an anonymous individual, we believe their concern is valid.

3.4 Prenatal testing

Even though it is rarely requested, prenatal testing has raised a few concerns. Although few clinical service laboratories maintain the ability to assay markers linked to the HD gene since the advent of a direct gene test, occasional patients still opt for exclusion testing but have difficulty finding a laboratory to provide the desired service. The dearth of reports documenting successful application of preimplantation genetic diagnosis techniques to this particular disorder, and the high cost and limited availability of the procedure in the US has been a concern to some patients and counsellors. Finally, complex counselling situations occasionally arise in the context of prenatal testing. Two brief examples illustrate this point.

In the first case, a 42-year-old woman whose at-risk husband did not want to know his gene status requested fetal testing for both HD and Down's syndrome, and after a lengthy discussion with the genetic counsellor, offered a compromise in which the counsellor should do both tests and just tell her that 'something is wrong with the baby' if any abnormalities were detected, without revealing what the abnormality was. The husband was unwilling to participate in counselling.

In the second case, a woman in her late 20s whose sample had already been obtained by another physician came for the first time to a genetic counsellor to receive prenatal test results. The at-risk father of the fetus, who was not the patient's husband, did not want to know his gene status. The patient was in the process of divorcing her husband, which necessitated a change in healthcare providers and thus a new genetic counsellor.

Both of these cases illustrate the conflicts that can arise between a pregnant woman and an at-risk father of the fetus. Each case requires careful thought and sensitive counselling, and involved counsellors benefit from discussion with others who have had similar cases.

3.5 Predictive testing by non-specialists

Some patients in the US obtain predictive tests outside of predictive testing centres. Without complete reporting from both the laboratories and the predictive testing centres, it is impossible to quantify how often this occurs, or to what extent there are problems associated with predictive testing outside of defined predictive testing centres. In the US, patients who choose to use their medical insurance to pay for the testing procedure may be required by their insurer to undergo testing through the local neurologist or genetic counsellor, even if that person lacks experience with HD or with predictive testing. Laboratory directors struggle with whether, or to what extent, they should play a 'gatekeeper' role, by questioning or refusing to test samples that come from physicians who appear not to have provided for their patients the type or extent of counselling recommended in the IHA or HDSA guidelines. As genetic testing volume has increased, a number of laboratories have abandoned the role of gatekeeper; some send educational packets to testing physicians, whereas others advertise directly to neurologists and test without question whatever samples arrive in the laboratory. Education of neurologists and other physicians about genetic testing is necessary, and is one of the goals of the recently formed Neurogenetics Section of the American Academy of Neurology. At the same time, both the Huntington Disease Society of America, and the International Huntington Association are currently revising their 1994 Genetic testing guidelines.

3.6 Insurance problems

Concern about potential insurance discrimination is commonly cited as a reason for the relatively low uptake of predictive testing in the US compared with that in other countries. The actual number of people who have lost or been denied insurance on the basis of a gene test result to date appears to be quite low, and legislation has been written in many states to prevent medical insurers from having access to genetic test results. About 10% of at-risk individuals report problems with insurance even without genetic testing, presumably because of their at-risk status (Kallenborn, 1997). This is an area of ongoing surveillance by lay organizations, the US HD GTG and the AMDTG, because the growing number of individuals undergoing predictive gene tests for adult-onset disorders of any type have an ongoing potential for insurance discrimination, including many forms of insurance besides health insurance.

3.7 Other counselling issues

Predictive genetic testing continues to present unique challenges to its practitioners. Almqvist and her colleagues at the University of British Columbia found, in an ambitious worldwide survey, that the risk of psychiatric hospitalization, suicide attempt or successful suicide following genetic testing was quite low (Almqvist et al., 1999), perhaps confirming the impression of Codori et al. (1994) that those who choose to be tested are by and large psychologically equipped to adapt to the results, or perhaps demonstrating that the genetic and psychological counselling that predictive testing centres provide is beneficial. However, recalling earlier admonitions that HD affects a broader audience than just the patient (Burgess, 1994; Kessler, 1993), several recent reports have focused on the significant and sometimes negative effects of predictive testing on other family members, and even on the friend or companion who accompanies the tested individual to clinic appointments (Jacobs and Deatrick, 1999; Quaid and Wesson, 1995; Sobel and Cowan, 2000; Williams et al., 2000). For some patients, adjusting to normal results presents a challenge (Williams et al., 2000). And, although the risk of severe adverse consequences is low, the long-term effects of testing positive can include increases in anxiety and depression and a decrease in self-esteem (Taylor and Myers, 1997).

4. The contribution of predictive testing populations to research

One consequence of predictive testing is the subdivision of the at-risk population, whereas previously HD family members were either affected or at-risk, now there are affected, at-risk-not-tested, at-risk known gene carriers and formerly-at-risk non-gene carriers. In addition to their obvious contribution to the study of predictive testing itself, these groups form an attractive pool of potential clinical research subjects.

In a pivotal study, CAG repeat data from over one thousand affected and at-risk individuals were incorporated in a life-table analysis of age of disease onset (Brinkman *et al.*, 1997). Although clinicians remain divided about how or whether to incorporate the results of this study in clinical practice, it was the first step in the development of a new algorithm for determining onset age in HD, which will likely be an important tool in the design of future clinical trials.

Others have begun to look critically at serial neurologic examination and neuroimaging features of presymptomatic gene carriers, in order to define disease onset more accurately, which will be critical in future clinical trials of putative preventive or disease-delaying therapies (Harris *et al.*, 1999; Kirkwood *et al.*, 2000). The Huntington Study Group, a University of Rochester (NY)-led international consortium of clinical trials centres, has embarked on a large-scale longitudinal observational assessment of non-gene tested at-risk individuals (under the acronym, PHAROS), in order to define clinical features of disease onset, free of investigator or subject bias. A companion study of known HD gene carriers called PREDICT-HD, using more invasive evaluations such as neuroimaging or neuropsychometric assessment, will lead to a much better understanding of the years immediately preceding and culminating in the development of overt HD.

Research utilizing the at-risk or gene-positive populations must be undertaken with caution and an appreciation of all the ethical, legal and social concerns that accompany the predictive testing process. To date, the existence of observational studies does not seem to have increased the number of at-risk individuals seeking predictive genetic testing. However, once a disease-delaying or modifying therapy is identified, it will likely be of interest to study the treatment in a presymptomatic population. There is a great potential for the genetic testing floodgates to open at that point, with at-risk individuals who would not otherwise undergo testing requesting a test in the hope of getting access to an experimental therapy. Design of any therapeutic trial in the at-risk or gene-positive populations must be considered very carefully, to avoid the possibility of coercing patients into predictive testing or participation in the trial.

5. Conclusions

The era of 'predictive medicine' has begun, ushered in by pioneers in neurogenetics. The potential effects of predictive test results on patients, their families and acquaintances, continue to demand careful forethought by patients and genetics professionals. The very real potential for therapeutic trials in the at-risk populations within a short number of years is exciting, but at the same time humbling. We believe that professional consortia provide a useful environment for discussion and improvement of clinical practice in this area, as well as a mechanism for maintaining the broad overview necessary to foster useful interactions with lay groups, non-genetics physicians, and clinical and basic science researchers.

References

Adam, S., Wiggins, S., Whyte, P., *et al.* (1993) Five year study of prenatal testing for Huntington's disease: demand, attitudes, and psychological assessment. *J. Med. Genet.* **30:** 549–556.

Almqvist, E.W., Bloch, M., Brinkman, R., Craufurd, D. and Hayden, M.R. (1999) A worldwide assessment of the frequency of suicide, suicide attempts, or psychiatric hospitalization after predictive testing for Huntington disease. *Am. J. Hum. Genet.* **64:** 1293–1304.

Alonso, M.E., Rescas, P., Cisneros, B., Martinez, C., Silva, G., Ochoa, A. and Montanez, C. (1997) Analysis of the (CAG)n repeat causing Huntington's disease in a Mexican population. *Clin. Genet.* **51:** 225–230.

Alonso Vilatela, M.E., Ochoa Morales, A., Garcia de la Cadena, C., Ruiz Lopez, I., Marinez Aranda, C. and Villa, A. (1999) Predictive and prenatal diagnosis of Huntington's disease: attitudes of Mexican neurologists, psychiatrists, and psychologists. *Arch. Med. Res.* **30:** 320–324.

American College of Medical Genetics/American Society of Human Genetics Huntington Disease Genetic Testing Working Group (1998) Laboratory guidelines for Huntington disease genetic testing. *Am. J. Hum. Genet.* **62:** 1243–1247.

American Society of Human Genetics Board of Directors and the American College of Medical Genetics Board of Directors (1995) Points to consider: ethical, legal, and psychosocial implications of genetic testing in children and adolescents. *Am. J. Hum. Genet.* **57:** 1233–1241.

Andrew, S.E., Goldberg, Y.P., Theilmann, J., Zeisler, J. and Hayden, M.R. (1994) A CCG repeat polymorphism adjacent to the CAG repeat in the Huntington disease gene: implications for diagnostic accuracy and predictive testing. *Hum. Mol. Genet.* **3:** 65–67.

Anonymous (1994) Guidelines for the molecular genetics predictive test in Huntington's disease. *Neurology* **44:** 1533–1536.

Babul, R., Adam, S., Kremer, B., Dufresne, S., Wiggins, S., Huggins, M., Theilmann, J., Bloch, M. and Hayden, M.R. (1993) Attitudes toward direct predictive testing for the Huntington disease gene. Relevance for other adult-onset disorders. The Canadian Collaborative Group on Predictive Testing for Huntington Disease. *JAMA* **270:** 2321–2325.

Benjamin, C.M., Adam, S., Wiggins, S., *et al.* (1994) Proceed with care: direct predictive testing for Huntington disease. *Am. J. Hum. Genet.* **55:** 606–617.

Braude, P.R., De Wert, G.M., Evers Kiebooms, G., Pettigrew, R.A. and Geraedts, J.P. (1998) Non-disclosure preimplantation genetic diagnosis for Huntington's disease: practical and ethical dilemmas. *Prenatal Diagn.* **18:** 1422–1426.

Brinkman, R.R., Mezei, M.M., Theilmann, J., Almqvist, E. and Hayden, M.R. (1997) The likelihood of being affected with Huntington disease by a particular age, for a specific CAG repeat size. *Am. J. Hum. Genet.* **60:** 1202–1210.

Burgess, M.M. (1994) Ethical issues in prenatal testing. *Clin. Biochem.* **27:** 87–91.

Burgess, M.M., Adam, S., Bloch, M. and Hayden, M.R. (1998) Dilemmas of anonymous predictive testing for Huntington disease: privacy vs. optimal care. *Am. J. Med. Genet.* **71:** 197–201.

Codori, A.M. and Brandt, J. (1994) Psychological costs and benefits of predictive testing for Huntington's disease. *Am. J. Med. Genet.* **54:** 174–184.

Codori, A.M., Hanson, R. and Brandt, J. (1994) Self-selection in predictive testing for Huntington's disease. *Am. J. Med. Genet.* **54:** 167–173.

Copley, T.T., Wiggins, S., Dufrasne, S., Bloch, M., Adam, S., McKellin, W. and Harper PS, Lim C, Craufurd D, on behalf of the UK Huntington's Disease Prediction Consortium. (2000) Ten years of presymptomatic testing for Huntington's disease: the experience of the UK Huntington's Disease Prediction Consortium. *J Med Genet* **37:** 567–571.

Harris, G.J., Codori, A.M., Lewis, R.F., Schmidt, E., Bedi, A. and Brandt, J. (1999) Reduced basal ganglia blood flow and volume in pre-symptomatic, gene-tested persons at-risk for Huntington's disease. *Brain* **122:** 1667–1678.

Hayden, M.R. (1995) Are we all of one mind? Clinicians' and patients' opinions regarding the development of a service protocol for predictive testing for Huntington disease. Canadian Collaborative Study for Predictive Testing for Huntington Disease. *Am. J. Med. Genet.* **58:** 59–69.

Hayden, M.R., Bloch, M. and Wiggins, S. (1995) Psychological effects of predictive testing for Huntington's disease. *Adv. Neurol.* **65:** 201–210.

Huntington's Disease Society of America (2001) *Guidelines for Genetic Testing for Huntington's Disease.* Huntington's Disease Society of America Inc., New York.

Jacobs, L.A. and Deatrick, J.A. (1999) The individual, the family, and genetic testing. *J. Prof. Nursing* **15:** 313–324.

Kallenborn, M.M. (1997) A retrospective survey of attitudes toward presymptomatic testing for Huntington disease. Thesis, University of Pittsburgh.

Kessler, S. (1993) Forgotten person in the Huntington disease family. *Am. J. Med. Genet.* **48:** 145–150.

Kirkwood, S.C., Siemers, E., Bond, C., Conneally, P.M., Christian, J.C. and Foroud, T. (2000) Confirmation of subtle motor changes among presymptomatic carriers of the Huntington disease gene. *Arch. Neurol.* **57:** 1040–1044.

Lawson, K., Wiggins, S., Green, T., Adam, S., Bloch, M. and Hayden, M.R. (1996) Adverse psychological events occurring in the first year after predictive testing for Huntington's disease: the Canadian collaborative study predictive testing. *J. Med. Genet.* **33:** 856–862.

Nance, M.A., Mathias-Hagen, V., Breningstall, G., Wick, M.J. and McGlennan, R.C. (1999) Molecular diagnostic analysis of a very large trinucelotide repeat in a patient with juvenile Huntington disease. *Neurology* **52:** 392–394.

Nance, M.A., Myers, R.H. and the US Huntington Disease Genetic Testing Group (1999) Trends in predictive and prenatal testing for Huntington disease, 1993–1998. *Am. J. Hum. Genet.* **65 (Suppl.):** A406.

Nance, M.A. and the US Huntington Disease Genetic Testing Group (1997) Genetic testing of children at risk for Huntington's disease. *Neurology* **49:** 1048–1053.

Potter, N.T., Nance, M.A. for the Ataxia Molecular Diagnostic Testing Group (1998) Genetic testing for ataxia in North America. *Am. J. Hum. Genet.* **63:** A239.

Potter, N.T., Nance, M.A. for the Ataxia Molecular Diagnostic Testing Group (2000) Genetic testing for ataxia in North America. *Mol. Diagn.* **5:** 91–99.

Quaid, K.A. and Wesson, M.K. (1995) Exploration of the effects of predictive testing for Huntington disease on intimate relationships. *Am. J. Med. Genet.* **57:** 46–51.

Schulman, J.D. and Black, S.H. (1997) Screening for Huntington disease and certain other dominantly inherited disorders: a case for preimplantation genetic testing. *J. Med. Screen.* **4:** 58–59.

Schulman, J.D., Black, S.H., Handyside, A. and Nance, W.E. (1996) Preimplantation genetic testing for Huntington disease and certain other dominantly inherited disorders. *Clin. Genet.* **49:** 57–58.

Sharpe, N.F. (1994) Informed consent and Huntington disease: a model for communication. *Am. J. Med. Genet.* **50:** 239–246.

Sobel, S.K. and Cowan, D.B. (2000) Impact of genetic testing for Huntington disease on the family system. *Am. J. Med. Genet.* **90:** 49–59.

Stern, H.J., Harton, G.L., Sisson, M.E., Jones, S.L., Fallon, L.A., Thorsell, L.P., Getlinger, M.E., Black, S.H. and Schulman J.D. (2000). Non-disclosing preimplantation genetic diagnosis for Huntington disease *Am. J. Hum. Genet.* **67 (Suppl.):** A42.

Taylor, C.A. and Myers, R.H. (1997) Long-term impact of Huntington disease linkage testing. *Am. J. Med. Genet.* **70:** 365–370.

Uhlmann, W.R., Ginsburg, D., Gelehrter, T.D., Nicholson, J. and Petty, E.M. (1996) Questioning the need for anonymous genetic counseling and testing. *Am. J. Hum. Genet.* **59:** 968–970.

Visintainer, C.L., Matthias-Hagen, V. and Nance, M.A. for the US Huntington Disease Genetic Testing Group (2001) Anonymous predictive testing for Huntington's disease in the United States. *Genet. Test.* **5:** 213–218.

Wick, M.J., Matthias-Hagen, V.L., Allingham-Hawkins, D.J., Nance, M.A., Potter, N.T. for the Ataxia Molecular Diagnostic Testing Group (1999) Genetic testing for Friedreich ataxia. *Am. J. Hum. Genet.* **165:** A412.

Williams, J.K., Schutte, D.L., Evers, C. and Holkup, P.A. (2000) Redefinition: coping with normal results from predictive gene testing for neurodegenerative disorders. *Res. Nurs. Health* **23:** 260–269.

Williams, J.K., Schutte, D.L., Holkup, P.A., Evers, C. and Muilenberg, A. (2000) Psychosocial impact of predictive testing for Huntington disease on support persons. *Am. J. Med. Genet.* **96:** 353–359.

14

Conclusion
Prenatal testing for late-onset genetic disorders: evidence and insights from Huntington's disease

Peter S. Harper

1. Background

Prenatal genetic diagnosis has been feasible for over 30 years, initially based on chromosomal or enzymatic analysis for disorders such as Down's syndrome or Tay Sachs disease, but now feasible for a wide range of Mendelian conditions using molecular techniques. Originally only possible in mid-pregnancy through amniocentesis, the development of early (10–12 weeks) chorion villus sampling has greatly reduced the delays in obtaining a result, especially in those high-risk genetic situations in which the slightly greater risk of the procedure to the pregnancy may be a less critical factor.

From its origins to the present, prenatal diagnosis has been developed and applied principally in relation to genetic disorders that are largely untreatable, which cause severe physical and/or mental disability, and which have their onset at birth or in early life. This is entirely understandable and has reflected the demand for testing in pregnancy from parents where such disorders have occurred, or are at high risk of doing so, as well as the fact that this has been the main group in which prenatal diagnosis has been technically feasible.

This situation is now changing, at least from a technological viewpoint, as the identification of the genes underlying the majority of Mendelian disorders, together with a shared basis of molecular analysis, means that accurate

Prenatal Testing for Late-Onset Neurogenetic Diseases, edited by G. Evers-Kiebooms, M. W. Zoeteweij and P. S. Harper
©2002 BIOS Scientific Publishers Ltd, Oxford

prediction of disease is now potentially possible for all single gene disorders, regardless of age at onset or body systems affected. Although there remain important issues of clinical variability, gene penetrance and heterogeneity of mutations and genetic loci, these do not alter the basic situation that essentially all single gene disorders are, or are likely to become, prenatally predictable.

Whether this radical technological shift is, or is likely to be, paralleled by a corresponding increase in demand for prenatal testing in late-onset genetic disorders, is quite a different matter. To date, there are few signs that this is the case, and this provides both the opportunity and the urgent need for collecting evidence that will document the wishes, needs and attitudes of patients and families involved, as well as how clinical practice in this field is evolving. Until now this evidence is largely lacking, something which the collected chapters of this book provide a first, albeit preliminary step to remedying.

The group of inherited brain degenerations, of which Huntington's disease (HD) can be regarded as prototype (Harper, 1996), provides a particularly important group for which the subject of prenatal testing can be examined. Few would question the severity of the group, often with a combination of progressive physical and mental disability, producing a major burden for both patient and wider family. Currently, they are largely untreatable, though recent research advances offer the hope that this might change in the not too distant future. As a group, the disorders mostly follow clear (usually dominant) Mendelian inheritance, with a 50% risk to offspring of either sex of inheriting the condition; in a few instances (e.g.: familial Alzheimer's or motor neurone disease) the Mendelian cases form a rare subset of a much more frequent and largely sporadic wider group.

Finally, these conditions are late onset, rarely causing symptoms before adult life and occurring most frequently in middle life or even in old age. The well-recognized exceptions (e.g. juvenile HD) are too rare to affect this overall pattern. Add to this the fact that this group of inherited neurodegenerations has been a major focus of both demand and study in relation to genetic counselling and, more recently, predictive genetic testing, and it can be seen why the group is particularly appropriate for detailed analysis in relation to prenatal genetic testing.

Huntington's disease was the first autosomal dominant disease whose chromosomal location was accurately mapped by molecular techniques (Gusella et al., 1983) and the first approaches to prenatal prediction were reported in 1987 by Hayden et al. and Quarrell et al. Because direct molecular detection of the mutation, in adults or in pregnancy, was not detectable, these reports were of 'exclusion testing', allowing prediction of whether the pregnancy had received from the at-risk partner a low risk genotype (from the unaffected grandparent) or a high-risk (but not definitively abnormal) genotype from the affected grandparent. Direct prenatal prediction using linked markers was also used in suitably structured families (Maat-Kievit et al., 1999), but exclusion testing remained the most frequent approach in subsequent series (e.g. Tyler et al., 1990) until after the HD gene and mutation had been isolated (Huntington's Disease Collaborative Research Group, 1993).

Both presymptomatic and prenatal prediction had been the subject of widespread discussion and surveys before either became feasible and it is relevant that a considerable proportion of those asked stated that they would request prenatal testing in a future pregnancy, between 40 and 50% in surveys in Canada (Adam *et al.*, 1993) and Germany (Chapter 5), with even higher levels for the planned uptake of presymptomatic testing (see Harper *et al.*, 1996, for summary). As will be seen, the actual experience has proved to be very different. In all studies of the reasons why people have sought presymptomatic testing, reproductive decision-making has also been prominent (Decruyenaere *et al.*, 1995; Meissen *et al.*, 1991).

2. The evidence

Until the present collaborative study, evidence on the uptake and application of prenatal testing in HD has been scanty and for other inherited neurological degenerations virtually absent. Numerical data have been reported for Canada (Adam *et al.*, 1993), The Netherlands (Maat-Kievit *et al.*, 1999) and UK (Simpson and Harper, 2001) but only the Canadian and The Netherlands studies attempted to put the experience into the context of prediction and genetic counselling overall. From these studies it was already clear that prenatal testing in HD was relatively infrequent, so that a collaborative study involving several major centres would be needed to gain a comprehensive picture.

The six European countries involved in this study contain a little over 200 million people and are likely to have an approximately comparable population frequency of HD (Harper, 1992). The simple core data available for this large population, based on 305 pregnancies undergoing testing, greatly exceed any previously available, or indeed any likely to be available in future, whereas the seven individual centres were able to provide detailed information which simple surveys could never hope to obtain. Although the full data are given in the specific chapters, it is worth examining the key facts in this conclusion.

The first striking fact requiring consideration is that the six countries of the study fall into two groups, with the uptake of prenatal diagnosis in Belgium, The Netherlands and the UK being an order of magnitude higher than in France, Greece and Italy, the last country being to some extent intermediate (Chapter 3). The possible factors involved in this difference will be returned to (and are also raised in individual chapters) but the pattern is reinforced by the ancillary data provided from countries outside the primary study, with Denmark corresponding closely to the first group, whereas Germany, Austria, Switzerland and the USA (Chapter 13) conform to the second.

Do such 10-fold differences reflect the true needs and wishes of the populations involved? To what extent do they reflect inadequacies of coordinated data collection, or of public awareness, attitudes of professionals, availability and equitable access to health services? Are these data for HD likely to reflect future patterns for other late-onset disorders? It is impossible to answer these questions at present, but the important fact is that only the major dataset represented by the present study would have been able to identify these issues and to point out the need for further work.

An allied finding to emerge is that for the four 'high-uptake' countries (including Denmark), the use of prenatal diagnosis is rather uniform in frequency, both in absolute terms and in relation to the uptake of presymptomatic testing, with an approximate ratio of 10 : 1 for presymptomatic to prenatal tests. There seems to be no clear trend of increasing (or decreasing) uptake, and it is of interest that exclusion testing has remained a significant option (one-third of the total prenatal tests) even when specific prediction is feasible (Simpson and Harper, 2001), clearly indicating the importance that couples attach to their wish to know (or not to know) parental status, alongside their wish to have a child free from the risk of HD.

A strength of the present dataset is that it has clearly shown that predictive testing does influence subsequent reproductive outcomes and uptake of prenatal testing. This was only possible because the study chose to analyse the wider area of predictive tests rather than to restrict the data to pregnancy alone and it has allowed what is probably the most important conclusion to emerge (Chapter 4). For the 451 individuals with predictive test results studied, there had been 442 pregnancies before the individuals knew their carrier status, 388 ending in liveborn children, with 22 terminations. When this group became separated into known mutation carriers (180) and non-carriers (271) the pregnancy rate of non-carriers was more than twice that of carriers, the differential being maintained in the subgroup for whom reproductive reasons were stated as particularly important for having predictive testing. Overall, in the 142 pregnancies occurring after presymptomatic testing, 142 children were born (111 known to be free from the risk of HD either as a result of parental or pregnancy testing) with only 16 terminations.

These results are the first to give information in any late-onset genetic disorder on the inter-relationship between prenatal and presymptomatic testing and reproductive outcomes and clearly show the value of examining prenatal testing in its wider context. It is most unlikely that such a clear pattern could have emerged from the smaller population bases of individual centres and this reinforces the value of collaborative studies when these issues are analysed in other types of disorder.

Other points emerge with clarity from the combined dataset, notably that prenatal diagnosis was rarely requested when the parent was affected by HD (this occurred mainly in the UK sample), the great majority of parents being either at risk, or known mutation carriers. Again this indicates that couples make their decisions in the broader context, including whether a parent's health is likely to allow the caring for a child.

Before leaving the quantitative evidence base, it must be recognized that some of the key evidence needed was not, and could not be collected, yet it is vital if we are to obtain a true picture. What about those families, considering or during a pregnancy, who are never referred to a genetics centre but are dealt with by primary care physicians, neurologists or obstetricians? Do they receive the same full and objective support as do most families managed by geneticists? Are the reproductive outcomes, including termination of pregnancy, comparable with those recorded in the present study? Anecdotal and personal experience suggests that this is far from always being the case. Yet only in a minority of countries are medical genetic services for adult genetic disorders well developed and comprehensive (Harris *et al.*, 1998), so what is recorded here may represent a pattern closer to optimal care than what is generally the norm.

The quantitative data of the European Collaborative Study have provided firm foundations on which some preliminary conclusions can be based and which can point to further work that is needed. But this only represents one aspect of the information available and its quantitative aspect can easily blunt or mask many of the key factors that we need to recognize and understand, especially the individual and personal ones. To see this important side we need to look at the case histories involving prenatal (and preimplantation) testing and the lessons that these can teach us.

3. The personal perspective: individual case histories

The two groups of case histories contained in this book are of irreplaceable value; it would be seriously incomplete without them and would lose a special quality of relevance and individual involvement. Anyone working outside this field who reads them can see immediately why this book is needed and important, and how great the impact of the disorder and the associated issues, genetic and other, are to the individuals involved. For those of us already closely involved with patients and families, one can immediately recognize similar cases that one has been personally associated with. It is not just the gravity, but the complexity and sensitivity of the issues that make an impact on the reader, along with the variability of response by different people placed in what might, at first glance, appear comparable situations. The effects of family structures and relationships, and of individual personalities is evident. One cannot but feel both compassion and respect for the individuals and their partners, trying their best to overcome successive difficulties in what at times seem impossible situations; one wonders how one would cope oneself if confronted in one's own life by such problems? The same respect is felt for those counsellors and psychologists involved who have told the stories with such sensitivity and who have undoubtedly provided invaluable support.

These difficult issues have always existed for HD families, long before prenatal or predictive testing was feasible, but has one really helped by adding the complexities of molecular technology to an already fraught situation? I suspect that it would be easy to identify specific cases where this had indeed helped, but also others where it had harmed; perhaps the latter are more likely to be found where a family has not had the support of skilled professionals as in the cases described here. Very real questions are raised by the authors as to whether families can become trapped by technology, especially in the face of a series of consecutive adverse results; who could imagine when setting out on this road that they might have up to five successive abnormal results – and who as a professional could imagine that a couple would survive such an experience?

The experiences given in this collection of case histories go some way to explain why workers on HD often show such a loyalty to working on the disorder, whether they are clinicians, laboratory workers or social scientists. The shared experience has helped to create a community of workers whose links outlast shifts in technology.

The case reports have, however, a value greater than their emotional impact; they point to the development of a further category of evidence, largely qualitative in nature, that can use the approaches of the social sciences, psychotherapy and linguistics to extract material from the individual interview which can be objectively analysed, and in turn used to improve clinical practice. Although such approaches were not part of the European Collaboration itself, the study and, in particular, the specific case histories, provide the spur to setting up the frameworks that can develop this different type of evidence. Again, however, some of the evidence one needs is likely to be the most elusive; how, for instance, could one capture the experiences of those involved in prenatal or predictive testing who had never had access to skilled professionals when considering or undergoing such tests?

4. The legal, ethical and social framework

Early prenatal genetic diagnosis only entered clinical practice to a significant extent when changes in the law legalized termination of pregnancy in situations of high risk for a disorder in the fetus. These changes were (and in some countries still are) accompanied by considerable public debate and prenatal and preimplantation diagnosis still remains a sensitive and controversial area. Thus, the specific chapters on legal and ethical aspects of prenatal diagnosis for late-onset genetic disorders (Chaters 6 and 9) are of considerable importance in providing a framework within which clinical practice can develop.

As the chapters make clear, the legal aspects in particular were framed in the context of early-onset genetic disorders and the issues for those of later onset have been largely reserved for professional discussions. Thus, the situation in relation to HD and comparable disorders largely turns on the question of whether the absence of statements relating to late-onset disorders in the various laws precludes termination after prenatal testing, or whether it allows the practice in what may be considered reasonable circumstances. It is reassuring for a non-lawyer to find that the latter is largely the case, and that the practice of a particular field of medicine to high and accepted professional standards is not likely to be undermined by technical legal niceties. It is also a surprise to realize how little actual 'case law' there is in the field, and somewhat sobering to see how much importance legal experts attach to 'guidelines', or even to a less than fully considered statement that one happens to have set down in print in the past!

The ethical issues likewise seem to turn around what as a non-expert one might consider 'real life' or 'practice-based' issues, which is reassuring. Perhaps the European project consciously (or subconsciously) chose ethical and legal experts for the study who think comparably with ordinary people! In any event, it would seem accepted that prenatal testing for severe and untreatable late-onset genetic disorders need not be ruled out simply because they are of late onset. It will be of great interest in future to examine the ethical issues in the context of individual case histories; not as a hurdle or obstacle for particular families, but because there are likely to be many lessons to be learned from particular examples that may not emerge clearly from an overall series.

Prenatal and predictive testing for HD and related disorders is profoundly influenced by the wider family and social context. In this respect the choice of centres from different parts of Europe might have been expected to show considerable differences, but this was not really so, except in the distinction, already mentioned, that Southern Europe generally showed a marked lower uptake of prenatal testing. However, it is difficult, even in the most preliminary way, to attribute this difference to the overall structure of society; perhaps a series of social factors are involved. Thus, Greece, where prenatal testing for HD is minimal, has a long history of widespread use of prenatal diagnosis for haemoglobinopathies, coordinated as a national screening programme; it is suggested that the fact of HD being mainly handled by neurologists, and the weakness of clinical genetics as a speciality, could be relevant factors (Chapter 5). Similarly, the low uptake of prenatal testing in Germany, in comparison with the comparable societies of Belgium and The Netherlands, seems puzzling until one remembers the experience of HD families under the Third Reich (see Harper, 1996, Chapter 11), likely to be a potent factor still today. Finally, why should uptake be so low in the USA (Chapter 13)? Is this a lack of full coordinated data across the country, or does it reflect the structure and need to pay for medical services; itself an important factor in social structure?

An important barometer in how new services are being delivered is provided by lay societies, with whom HD professionals have a long tradition of close collaboration. It is they, rather than expert centres, that are best able to provide case histories showing where things have gone badly wrong and perhaps they could provide the starting point for future qualitative studies. Unfortunately, for HD at least, such societies tend to be weakest in those countries whose medical and genetic services are also least developed, whose voice is less heard when the European experience is being reported.

5. Prenatal testing for late-onset disorders in clinical practice

The European Collaborative Study has clearly shown that prenatal testing for HD can only be considered meaningfully if it is analysed in the overall context, together with presymptomatic testing. The study illustrates clearly what previously had only been hinted at; reproductive and family plans are not only an important reason for presymptomatic testing but these to a large extent determine whether and how prenatal testing is used. Many couples, who might wish to undertake prenatal testing to achieve the aim of children free from the risk of HD, no longer have to do so because they have already had a normal presymptomatic test result.

Thus, the clinical practice of prenatal and presymptomatic testing needs to be closely coordinated, both forming part of the range of options associated with genetic counselling. Precisely which, if any, form of testing is taken up will depend on the nature, wishes and particular circumstances of the individuals involved, and may well vary with time. Clearly then it is better if the same professionals can be involved, who ideally may already know the couple and who should have had the opportunity to discuss the possibility and implications of prenatal testing before it is intended to embark on a pregnancy.

I suspect that it is only rarely that practitioners in other specialities than medical genetics have the experience, motivation, facilities and time to do this demanding task to a high standard. Fortunately, most obstetricians and neurologists recognize that this is not likely to be something they can take a lead role in, other than in the key aspect of the specific procedures. But what is the situation in those numerous countries in which medical genetics is poorly developed or orientated mainly to paediatric disorders? Again the present study is likely to reflect the practice mainly of expert centres and we need to know the overall picture.

The role of the molecular diagnostic laboratory is a vital one in the overall process and has perhaps been understated in this volume. Although the technical aspects of analysing prenatal samples have been largely resolved (Warner et al., 1993) and quality control schemes introduced, the need for close links between laboratory and clinical/counselling staff is as great as ever. These links are fortunately in place in most European centres and in Canada, but this seems to be far from being the case generally in USA, which stands in striking contrast in terms of overall clinical practice in this field.

The need for close coordination is at its greatest with preimplantation genetic diagnosis, in which the experience of the only two European centres established for this in Huntington's disease is reported (Chapter 7). Apart from a single American abstract report (Stern et al., 2000) there are no other published results, but one is frequently struck by the lack of awareness of the wider aspects of other centres proposing to become involved with late-onset disorders and by their reluctance to report details of preliminary research (including failures). It is profoundly to be hoped that all centres becoming involved in preimplantation diagnosis for late-onset genetic disorders will learn from the overall experience obtained in prenatal and presymptomatic testing for these conditions.

6. Huntington's disease as a model for other late-onset genetic disorders

Why is it that HD has been used so widely as a model for other late-onset disorders, not just those of the nervous system, but others such as muscle disorders and familial cancers? Indeed, should it be used as such a model? Some colleagues involved in other conditions seem to find it irritating that HD is always held up as the reference point! The fact remains, however, that HD continues to be the main model (although there is now a rapid growth of information on familial cancers) and that there are good reasons for this. It is worth examining these briefly.

The first reason is that HD was indeed the first, with presymptomatic and prenatal prediction becoming feasible through linked markers some years before it was possible for other late-onset genetic disorders. Second, the amount of practical experience has been much greater than for other neurological disorders, in which prenatal testing experience remains minimal and presymptomatic testing still limited. This is not simply the result of the relative prevalence of HD, but reflects also the fact that it is a disorder in which families have been seen for genetic counselling over many years, and where in a number of regions specific population studies and genetic registers have resulted in continuing contact being maintained.

A third reason for using HD as the prototype is that professionals and families have together evolved guidelines for clinical practice, starting from the earliest stages of predictive testing entering practice (World Federation of Neurology Research Group, 1993) and that, because the initial studies were undertaken in a research setting, we have a wealth of psychological as well as clinical data, from many different countries, though it has to be said that data on prenatal testing have, by comparison, been relatively deficient until the present study. A personal view I have long held is also that HD produces such a constellation of difficulties and challenges that if one can work out a reasonably successful model of practice for presymptomatic or prenatal prediction, it will probably also work for other disorders. Finally, the HD research community has always been highly collaborative in nature, allowing multicentre studies to obtain information that would be inadequate or impossible to draw conclusions from if confined to a single centre.

To date, no other group of late-onset disorders has matched this set of characteristics, nor is it likely that any other neurological late-onset disorders will do so. However, valuable information is now appearing for familial cancers, notably familial breast-ovarian cancer, which should help to identify the differences that result from the different organs involved and from the availability of at least some therapeutic options.

7. The future

There is little doubt that this field will see radical change, but which aspects are likely to be most altered? It could be argued that preimplantation diagnosis, with the avoidance of the need for termination, might largely replace prenatal testing for HD and other late-onset disorders. This seems unlikely in the near future, while the complexities, need for multiple procedures and modest current success rate means that it still has some way to go before it can be regarded as an established service, and yet further to go before it can be recommended outside the exceedingly few centres with an adequate track record.

A more likely change, in my view, may come from therapeutic initiatives in HD and in other progressive adult neurological disorders, which are now reaching the point of clinical trials. Whether the most successful approach proves to be neurotransplantation (Dunnett and Rosser, in press) or some pharmacological approach based on our increasing understanding of the pathogenesis, this is likely to have a major effect on attitudes to prediction, which could occur even if it is only the perception, rather than the proof of effectiveness that is accepted.

Such a change in perceived treatability of HD could well lead to a rapid increase in uptake of presymptomatic testing, but any effect on prenatal testing might be more complex. An increase in the number of recognized mutation carriers might mean that more would request prenatal testing, but if therapy were to be considered likely to be effective in future this might give an opposite trend. This points to a clear need for the ongoing monitoring of both prenatal and presymptomatic testing, and for accurate documentation of the reasons for requesting these, something which should be feasible, at least for simple data, in the major European centres and Canada. Again, such possible changes emphasize the need for prenatal and presymptomatic testing to be considered together.

The other likely, and to be hoped for, change is that HD will lose its present status as the overwhelming provider of data and that other late-onset disorders will emerge to give direct and coordinated results. This should help to determine which aspects of prenatal and presymptomatic testing are truly specific for HD or other individual conditions and which are more general; this will allow the basic principles and shared core aspects to be more accurately defined, as well as helping to evolve more specific patterns of practice appropriate to individual disorders.

It may be asked whether prenatal and predictive testing will become established for common late-onset disorders, neurological or other, which numerically far outweigh late-onset Mendelian disorders. The view has frequently been expressed, on the basis of minimal evidence, that such susceptibility testing will become commonplace in the near future and will largely supplant testing for single gene disorders as part of medical practice. To date, there are few signs of this happening, and although such a scenario is seductive to health planners of 'personalized medicine' (and to those with commercial interests in widespread genetic testing), it seems implausible and improbable in the near future. Not only are the specific genes involved in common disorders proving hard to find, they are also turning out, where identifiable, to be of small or minimal individual effect (except for the Mendelian subsets that can be dealt with as in other entirely Mendelian disorders). There is also increasing recognition of the complexity of interactions between different genes, rendering the concept of clear-cut identification of susceptibility unrealistic in most situations and difficult in all. Prenatal testing seems even less plausible for common polygenic disorders in the foreseeable future. Thus, we will probably have to continue to study Mendelian late-onset disorders as the basis for our understanding and clinical practice.

8. Conclusion

It is rare that a major multicentre study is able both to produce a large body of data on which important conclusions can be based and also to examine the more general issues involved, but the European Collaborative Study has probably achieved just this combination. The involvement of seven centres with closely similar approaches allowed the use of a common dataset that would have been impossible had the centres been working previously in entirely different ways. The fact that at least a core of data was obtainable from entire countries, representing a total population of over 200 million, gives a validity to the study that might have been lacking had it been confined to a single centre or country.

As with any successful study, the project has raised and recognized more questions than it has answered. Some of these will require longitudinal study in the light of evolving clinical practice and terminology; others will need a different set of approaches, using the wealth of existing and future case material seen so vividly in the case histories given in this book. Finally, the challenge has been offered to those working on other types of late-onset genetic disease to match and if possible surpass what the Huntington's research community has been able to achieve so far.

At present, the reproductive issues raised by serious late-onset genetic disorders remain a severe burden to those who are affected or at risk, and to their partners and family members. This study shows that through prenatal and presymptomatic testing, carried out in the context of skilled and sensitive genetic counselling, we have been able to be of some help to such families, even when they may opt not to pursue the actual testing options. There remain many for whom existing options are unsatisfactory, and probably many more worldwide who never have the opportunity to even consider them. We all need to work towards the situation in which the possibilities are not only improved for some families, but are available to all who need them. Whether families will in future be better able to be helped towards their goal of achieving their own family free from risk of serious disorder through prenatal or presymptomatic testing, through advances in therapy or through yet other approaches, remains to be seen; in the meantime this book, and the European Collaborative Study on which it is based, have provided a first step towards identifying the complexity of the factors involved and those patterns of practice that are most likely to help families and also most likely to avoid causing harm.

References

Adam, S., Wiggins, S., Whyte, P., *et al* (1993) Five year study of prenatal testing for Huntington's disease: demand, attitudes and psychological assessment. *J. Med. Genet.* **30:** 549–556.

Decruyenaere, M., Evers-Kiebooms, G., Boogaerts, A., Cassiman, J.-J., Cloostermans, T., Demyttenaere, K., Dom, R., Fryns, J.-P. and Van den Berghe, H. (1995) Predictive testing for Huntington's disease: risk perception, reasons for testing and psychological profile of test applicants. *Genet. Counsel.* **6:** 1–13.

Dunnett, S.B. and Rosser, A.E. (2002) Cell and tissue transplantation. In: *Huntington's Disease*, 3rd Edn (eds G. Bates. P.S. Harper and A.L. Jones) (in press).

Gusella, J.F., Wexler, N.S., Conneally, P.M., Naylor, S.L., Anderson, M.A., Tanzi, R.E., Watkins, P.C., Ottina, K., Wallace, M.R., Sakaguchi, A.Y., Young, A.B., Shoulson, I., Bonilla, E. and Martin J.B. (1983) A polymorphic DNA marker genetically linked to Huntington's disease. *Nature* 306: 234–238.

Harper, P.S. (1992) The epidemiology of Huntington's disease. *Hum. Genet.* 89: 365–376.

Harper, P.S. (ed) (1996) *Huntington's Disease*. Saunders, London.

Harper, P.S., Houlihan, G. and Tyler, A. (1996) Genetic counselling in Huntington's disease. In: *Huntington's Disease* (ed. P.S. Harper). Saunders, London, pp 359–393.

Hayden, M.R., Kastelein, J.J.P., Wilson, R.D., Hilbert, C., Hewit, J., Langlois, S., Fox, S. and Bloch, M. (1987) First trimester prenatal diagnosis for Huntington's disease with DNA probes. *Lancet* 1284–1285.

Huntington's Disease Collaborative Research Group (1993) A novel gene containing a trinucleotide repeat that is expanded and unstable on Huntington's disease chromosomes. *Cell* 72: 971–983.

Maat-Kievit A., Vegter-van der Vlis, M., Zoeteweij, M., Losekoot, M., van Haeringen, A., Kanhai, H. and Roos, R. (1999) Experience in prenatal testing for Huntington's disease in the Netherlands: procedures, results and guidelines (1987–1997). *Prenatal Diagn.* 19: 450–457.

Quarrell, O.W.J., Tyler, A., Meredith, A.L., Youngman, S., Upadhyaya, M. and Harper, P.S. (1987) Exclusion testing for Huntington's disease in pregnancy with a closely linked DNA marker. *Lancet* i: 1281–1283.

Simpson, S.A. and Harper, P.S. (2001) Prenatal testing for Huntington's disease: experience within the UK 1994–1998. *J. Med. Genet.* 38: 333–335.

Stern, H.J., Harton, G.L., Sisson, S.L. *et al.* (2000) Non-disclosing preimplantation genetic diagnosis for Huntington's disease. *Am. J. Hum. Genet.* 67 **(Suppl.):** 42 (abstract).

Tyler, A., Quarrell, O.W.J., Lazarou, L.P., Meredith, A.L. and Harper, P.S. (1990) Exclusion testing in pregnancy for Huntington's disease. *J. Med. Genet.* 27: 488–495.

Warner, J.P., Barron, L.H. and Brock, D.J. (1993) A new polymerase chain reaction (PCR) assay for the trinucleotide repeat that is unstable and expanded on Huntington's disease chromosomes. *Mol. Cell. Probes* 7: 235–239.

World Federation of Neurology Research Group on Huntington's Disease (1993) Presymptomatic testing for Huntington's disease: a world-wide survey. *J. Med. Genet.* 30: 1020–1022.

Index